AIR FRYER RECIPES 2021

EFFORTLESS DELICIOUS RECIPES FOR HEALTHIER FRIED

KIM BINAGHI

Table of Contents

Turkey, Peas and Mushrooms Casserole

Preparation time: 10 minutes **Cooking time:** 20 minutes
Servings: 4

Ingredients:

- 2 pounds turkey breasts, skinless, boneless
- Salt and black pepper to the taste
- 1 yellow onion, chopped
- 1 celery stalk, chopped
- ½ cup peas
- 1 cup chicken stock
- 1 cup cream of mushrooms soup
- 1 cup bread cubes

Directions:

1. In a pan that fits your air fryer, mix turkey with salt, pepper, onion, celery, peas and stock, introduce in your air fryer and cook at 360 degrees F for 15 minutes.
2. Add bread cubes and cream of mushroom soup, stir toss and cook at 360 degrees F for 5 minutes more.
3. Divide among plates and serve hot.

Enjoy!

Nutrition: calories 271, fat 9, fiber 9, carbs 16, protein 7

Tasty Chicken Thighs

Preparation time: 10 minutes **Cooking time:** 20 minutes
Servings: 6

Ingredients:

- 2 and ½ pounds chicken thighs
- Salt and black pepper to the taste
- 5 green onions, chopped
- 2 tablespoons sesame oil
- 1 tablespoon sherry wine
- ½ teaspoon white vinegar
- 1 tablespoon soy sauce
- ¼ teaspoon sugar

Directions:

1. Season chicken with salt and pepper, rub with half of the sesame oil, add to your air fryer and cook at 360 degrees F for 20 minutes.
2. Meanwhile, heat up a pan with the rest of the oil over medium high heat, add green onions, sherry wine, vinegar, soy sauce and sugar, toss, cover and cook for 10 minutes

3. Shred chicken using 2 forks divide among plates, drizzle sauce all over and serve.

Enjoy!

Nutrition: calories 321, fat 8, fiber 12, carbs 36, protein 24

Chicken Tenders and Flavored Sauce

Preparation time: 10 minutes **Cooking time:** 10 minutes
Servings: 6

Ingredients:

- 1 teaspoon chili powder
- 2 teaspoon garlic powder
- 1 teaspoon onion powder
- 1 teaspoon sweet paprika
- Salt and black pepper to the taste
- 2 tablespoons butter
- 2 tablespoons olive oil
- 2 pounds chicken tenders
- 2 tablespoons cornstarch
- ½ cup chicken stock
- 2 cups heavy cream
- 2 tablespoons water
- 2 tablespoons parsley, chopped

Directions:

1. In a bowl, mix garlic powder with onion powder, chili, salt, pepper and paprika, stir, add chicken and toss.

2. Rub chicken tenders with oil, place in your air fryer and cook at 360 degrees F for 10 minutes.
3. Meanwhile, heat up a pan with the butter over medium high heat, add cornstarch, stock, cream, water and parsley, stir, cover and cook for 10 minutes.
4. Divide chicken on plates, drizzle sauce all over and serve.

Enjoy!

Nutrition: calories 351, fat 12, fiber 9, carbs 20, protein 17

Duck and Veggies

Preparation time: 10 minutes **Cooking time:** 20 minutes

Servings: 8

Ingredients:

- 1 duck, chopped in medium pieces
- 3 cucumbers, chopped
- 3 tablespoon white wine
- 2 carrots, chopped
- 1 cup chicken stock
- 1 small ginger piece, grated
- Salt and black pepper to the taste

Directions:

1. In a pan that fits your air fryer, mix duck pieces with cucumbers, wine, carrots, ginger, stock, salt and pepper, toss, introduce in your air fryer and cook at 370 degrees F for 20 minutes.
2. Divide everything on plates and serve.

Enjoy!

Nutrition: calories 200, fat 10, fiber 8, carbs 20, protein 22

Chicken and Apricot Sauce

Preparation time: 10 minutes **Cooking time:** 20 minutes

Servings: 4

Ingredients:

- 1 whole chicken, cut into medium pieces
- Salt and black pepper to the taste
- 1 tablespoon olive oil
- ½ teaspoon smoked paprika
- ¼ cup white wine
- ½ teaspoon marjoram, dried
- ¼ cup chicken stock
- 2 tablespoons white vinegar
- ¼ cup apricot preserves
- 1 and ½ teaspoon ginger, grated
- 2 tablespoons honey

Directions:

1. Season chicken with salt, pepper, marjoram and paprika, toss to coat, add oil, rub well, place in your air fryer and cook at 360 degrees F for 10 minutes.

2. Transfer chicken to a pan that fits your air fryer, add stock, wine, vinegar, ginger, apricot preserves and honey, toss, put in your air fryer and cook at 360 degrees F for 10 minutes more.

3. Divide chicken and apricot sauce on plates and serve.

Enjoy!

Nutrition: calories 200, fat 7, fiber 19, carbs 20, protein 14

Chicken and Cauliflower Rice Mix

Preparation time: 10 minutes **Cooking time:** 20 minutes

Servings: 6

Ingredients:

- 3 bacon slices, chopped
- 3 carrots, chopped
- 3 pounds chicken thighs, boneless and skinless
- 2 bay leaves
- ¼ cup red wine vinegar
- 4 garlic cloves, minced
- Salt and black pepper to the taste
- 4 tablespoons olive oil
- 1 tablespoon garlic powder
- 1 tablespoon Italian seasoning
- 24 ounces cauliflower rice
- 1 teaspoon turmeric powder
- 1 cup beef stock

Directions:

1. Heat up a pan that fits your air fryer over medium high heat, add bacon, carrots, onion and garlic, stir and cook for 8 minutes.
2. Add chicken, oil, vinegar, turmeric, garlic powder, Italian seasoning and bay leaves, stir, introduce in your air fryer and cook at 360 degrees F for 12 minutes.
3. Add cauliflower rice and stock, stir, cook for 6 minutes more, divide among plates and serve.

Enjoy!

Nutrition: calories 340, fat 12, fiber 12, carbs 16, protein 8

Chicken and Spinach Salad

Preparation time: 10 minutes **Cooking time:** 12 minutes
Servings: 2

Ingredients:

- 2 teaspoons parsley, dried
- 2 chicken breasts, skinless and boneless
- ½ teaspoon onion powder
- 2 teaspoons sweet paprika
- ½ cup lemon juice
- Salt and black pepper to the taste
- 5 cups baby spinach
- 8 strawberries, sliced
- 1 small red onion, sliced
- 2 tablespoons balsamic vinegar
- 1 avocado, pitted, peeled and chopped
- ¼ cup olive oil
- 1 tablespoon tarragon, chopped

Directions:

1. Put chicken in a bowl, add lemon juice, parsley, onion powder and paprika and toss.

2. Transfer chicken to your air fryer and cook at 360 degrees F for 12 minutes.

3. In a bowl, mix spinach, onion, strawberries and avocado and toss.

4. In another bowl, mix oil with vinegar, salt, pepper and tarragon, whisk well, add to the salad and toss.

5. Divide chicken on plates, add spinach salad on the side and serve.

Enjoy!

Nutrition: calories 240, fat 5, fiber 13, carbs 25, protein 22

Chicken and Chestnuts Mix

Preparation time: 10 minutes **Cooking time:** 12 minutes
Servings: 2

Ingredients:

- ½ pound chicken pieces
- 1 small yellow onion, chopped
- 2 teaspoons garlic, minced
- A pinch of ginger, grated
- A pinch of allspice, ground
- 4 tablespoons water chestnuts
- 2 tablespoons soy sauce
- 2 tablespoons chicken stock
- 2 tablespoons balsamic vinegar
- 2 tortillas for serving

Directions:

1. In a pan that fits your air fryer, mix chicken meat with onion, garlic, ginger, allspice, chestnuts, soy sauce, stock and vinegar, stir, transfer to your air fryer and cook at 360 degrees F for 12 minutes.
2. Divide everything on plates and serve.

Nutrition: calories 301, fat 12, fiber 7, carbs 24, protein 12

Cider Glazed Chicken

Preparation time: 10 minutes **Cooking time:** 14 minutes

Servings: 4

Ingredients:

- 1 sweet potato, cubed
- 2 apples, cored and sliced
- 1 tablespoon olive oil
- 1 tablespoon rosemary, chopped
- Salt and black pepper to the taste
- 6 chicken thighs, bone in and skin on
- 2/3 cup apple cider
- 1 tablespoon mustard
- 2 tablespoons honey
- 1 tablespoon butter

Directions:

1. Heat up a pan that fits your air fryer with half of the oil over medium high heat, add cider, honey, butter and mustard, whisk well, bring to a simmer, take off heat, add chicken and toss really well.

2. In a bowl, mix potato cubes with rosemary, apples, salt, pepper and the rest of the oil, toss well and add to chicken mix.

3. Place pan in your air fryer and cook at 390 degrees F for 14 minutes.

4. Divide everything on plates and serve.

Enjoy!

Nutrition: calories 241, fat 7, fiber 12, carbs 28, protein 22

Veggie Stuffed Chicken Breasts

Preparation time: 10 minutes **Cooking time:** 15 minutes
Servings: 4

Ingredients:

- 4 chicken breasts, skinless and boneless
- 2 tablespoons olive oil
- Salt and black pepper to the taste
- 1 zucchini, chopped
- 1 teaspoon Italian seasoning
- 2 yellow bell peppers, chopped
- 3 tomatoes, chopped
- 1 red onion, chopped
- 1 cup mozzarella, shredded

Directions:

1. Mix a slit on each chicken breast creating a pocket, season with salt and pepper and rub them with olive oil.
2. In a bowl, mix zucchini with Italian seasoning, bell peppers, tomatoes and onion and stir.

3. Stuff chicken breasts with this mix, sprinkle mozzarella over them, place them in your air fryer's basket and cook at 350 degrees F for 15 minutes.
4. Divide among plates and serve.

Enjoy!

Nutrition: calories 300, fat 12, fiber 7, carbs 22, protein 18

Greek Chicken

Preparation time: 10 minutes **Cooking time:** 15 minutes

Servings: 4

Ingredients:

- 2 tablespoons olive oil
- Juice from 1 lemon
- 1 teaspoon oregano, dried
- 3 garlic cloves, minced
- 1 pound chicken thighs
- Salt and black pepper to the taste
- ½ pound asparagus, trimmed
- 1 zucchini, roughly chopped
- 1 lemon sliced

Directions:

1. In a heat proof dish that fits your air fryer, mix chicken pieces with oil, lemon juice, oregano, garlic, salt, pepper, asparagus, zucchini and lemon slices, toss, introduce in preheated air fryer and cook at 380 degrees F for 15 minutes.
2. Divide everything on plates and serve.

Enjoy!

Nutrition: calories 300, fat 8, fiber 12, carbs 20, protein 18

Duck Breasts with Red Wine and Orange Sauce

Preparation time: 10 minutes **Cooking time:** 35 minutes

Servings: 4

Ingredients:

- ½ cup honey
- 2 cups orange juice
- 4 cups red wine
- 2 tablespoons sherry vinegar
- 2 cups chicken stock
- 2 teaspoons pumpkin pie spice
- 2 tablespoons butter
- 2 duck breasts, skin on and halved
- 2 tablespoons olive oil
- Salt and black pepper to the taste

Directions:

1. Heat up a pan with the orange juice over medium heat, add honey, stir well and cook for 10 minutes.
2. Add wine, vinegar, stock, pie spice and butter, stir well, cook for 10 minutes more and take off heat.

3. Season duck breasts with salt and pepper, rub with olive oil, place in preheated air fryer at 370 degrees F and cook for 7 minutes on each side.
4. Divide duck breasts on plates, drizzle wine and orange juice all over and serve right away.

Enjoy!

Nutrition: calories 300, fat 8, fiber 12, carbs 24, protein 11

Duck Breast with Fig Sauce

Preparation time: 10 minutes **Cooking time:** 20 minutes

Servings: 4

Ingredients:

- 2 duck breasts, skin on, halved
- 1 tablespoon olive oil
- ½ teaspoon thyme, chopped
- ½ teaspoon garlic powder
- ¼ teaspoon sweet paprika
- Salt and black pepper to the taste
- 1 cup beef stock
- 3 tablespoons butter, melted
- 1 shallot, chopped
- ½ cup port wine
- 4 tablespoons fig preserves
- 1 tablespoon white flour

Directions:

1. Season duck breasts with salt and pepper, drizzle half of the melted butter, rub well, put in your air fryer's

basket and cook at 350 degrees F for 5 minutes on each side.

2. Meanwhile, heat up a pan with the olive oil and the rest of the butter over medium high heat, add shallot, stir and cook for 2 minutes.

3. Add thyme, garlic powder, paprika, stock, salt, pepper, wine and figs, stir and cook for 7-8 minutes.

4. Add flour, stir well, cook until sauce thickens a bit and take off heat.

5. Divide duck breasts on plates, drizzle figs sauce all over and serve.

Enjoy!

Nutrition: calories 246, fat 12, fiber 4, carbs 22, protein 3

Duck Breasts and Raspberry Sauce

Preparation time: 10 minutes **Cooking time:** 15 minutes

Servings: 4

Ingredients:

- 2 duck breasts, skin on and scored
- Salt and black pepper to the taste
- Cooking spray
- ½ teaspoon cinnamon powder
- ½ cup raspberries
- 1 tablespoon sugar
- 1 teaspoon red wine vinegar
- ½ cup water

Directions:

1. Season duck breasts with salt and pepper, spray them with cooking spray, put in preheated air fryer skin side down and cook at 350 degrees F for 10 minutes.

2. Heat up a pan with the water over medium heat, add raspberries, cinnamon, sugar and wine, stir, bring to a simmer, transfer to your blender, puree and return to pan.

3. Add air fryer duck breasts to pan as well, toss to coat, divide among plates and serve right away.

Enjoy!

Nutrition: calories 456, fat 22, fiber 4, carbs 14, protein 45

Duck and Cherries

Preparation time: 10 minutes **Cooking time:** 20 minutes

Servings: 4

Ingredients:

- ½ cup sugar
- ¼ cup honey
- 1/3 cup balsamic vinegar
- 1 teaspoon garlic, minced
- 1 tablespoon ginger, grated
- 1 teaspoon cumin, ground
- ½ teaspoon clove, ground
- ½ teaspoon cinnamon powder
- 4 sage leaves, chopped
- 1 jalapeno, chopped
- 2 cups rhubarb, sliced
- ½ cup yellow onion, chopped
- 2 cups cherries, pitted
- 4 duck breasts, boneless, skin on and scored
- Salt and black pepper to the taste

Directions:

1. Season duck breast with salt and pepper, put in your air fryer and cook at 350 degrees F for 5 minutes on each side.
2. Meanwhile, heat up a pan over medium heat, add sugar, honey, vinegar, garlic, ginger, cumin, clove, cinnamon, sage, jalapeno, rhubarb, onion and cherries, stir, bring to a simmer and cook for 10 minutes.
3. Add duck breasts, toss well, divide everything on plates and serve.

Enjoy!

Nutrition: calories 456, fat 13, fiber 4, carbs 64, protein 31

Easy Duck Breasts

Preparation time: 10 minutes **Cooking time:** 15 minutes
Servings: 4

Ingredients:

- 4 duck breasts, skinless and boneless
- 4 garlic heads, peeled, tops cut off and quartered
- 2 tablespoons lemon juice
- Salt and black pepper to the taste
- ½ teaspoon lemon pepper
- 1 and ½ tablespoon olive oil

Directions:

1. In a bowl, mix duck breasts with garlic, lemon juice, salt, pepper, lemon pepper and olive oil and toss everything.
2. Transfer duck and garlic to your air fryer and cook at 350 degrees F for 15 minutes.
3. Divide duck breasts and garlic on plates and serve.

Enjoy!

Nutrition: calories 200, fat 7, fiber 1, carbs 11, protein 17

Duck and Tea Sauce

Preparation time: 10 minutes **Cooking time:** 20 minutes

Servings: 4

Ingredients:

- 2 duck breast halves, boneless
- 2 and ¼ cup chicken stock
- ¾ cup shallot, chopped
- 1 and ½ cup orange juice
- Salt and black pepper to the taste
- 3 teaspoons earl gray tea leaves
- 3 tablespoons butter, melted
- 1 tablespoon honey

Directions:

1. Season duck breast halves with salt and pepper, put in preheated air fryer and cook at 360 degrees F for 10 minutes.
2. Meanwhile, heat up a pan with the butter over medium heat, add shallot, stir and cook for 2-3 minutes.
3. Add stock, stir and cook for another minute.
4. Add orange juice, tea leaves and honey, stir, cook for 2-3 minutes more and strain into a bowl.
5. Divide duck on plates, drizzle tea sauce all over and serve.

Enjoy!

Nutrition: calories 228, fat 11, fiber 2, carbs 20, protein 12

Marinated Duck Breasts

Preparation time: 1 day **Cooking time:** 15 minutes **Servings:** 2

Ingredients:
- 2 duck breasts
- 1 cup white wine
- ¼ cup soy sauce
- 2 garlic cloves, minced
- 6 tarragon springs
- Salt and black pepper to the taste
- 1 tablespoon butter
- ¼ cup sherry wine

Directions:
1. In a bowl, mix duck breasts with white wine, soy sauce, garlic, tarragon, salt and pepper, toss well and keep in the fridge for 1 day.
2. Transfer duck breasts to your preheated air fryer at 350 degrees F and cook for 10 minutes, flipping halfway.

3. Meanwhile, pour the marinade in a pan, heat up over medium heat, add butter and sherry, stir, bring to a simmer, cook for 5 minutes and take off heat.
4. Divide duck breasts on plates, drizzle sauce all over and serve.

Enjoy!

Nutrition: calories 475, fat 12, fiber 3, carbs 10, protein 48

Chicken Breasts with Passion Fruit Sauce

Preparation time: 10 minutes **Cooking time:** 10 minutes
Servings: 4

Ingredients:

- 4 chicken breasts
- Salt and black pepper to the taste
- 4 passion fruits, halved, deseeded and pulp reserved
- 1 tablespoon whiskey
- 2 star anise
- 2 ounces maple syrup
- 1 bunch chives, chopped

Directions:

1. Heat up a pan with the passion fruit pulp over medium heat, add whiskey, star anise, maple syrup and chives, stir well, simmer for 5-6 minutes and take off heat.
2. Season chicken with salt and pepper, put in preheated air fryer and cook at 360 degrees F for 10 minutes, flipping halfway.
3. Divide chicken on plates, heat up the sauce a bit, drizzle it over chicken and serve.

Enjoy!

Nutrition: calories 374, fat 8, fiber 22, carbs 34, protein 37

Chicken Breasts and BBQ Chili Sauce

Preparation time: 10 minutes **Cooking time:** 20 minutes

Servings: 6

Ingredients:

- 2 cups chili sauce
- 2 cups ketchup
- 1 cup pear jelly
- ¼ cup honey
- ½ teaspoon liquid smoke
- 1 teaspoon chili powder
- 1 teaspoon mustard powder
- 1 teaspoon sweet paprika
- Salt and black pepper to the taste
- 1 teaspoon garlic powder
- 6 chicken breasts, skinless and boneless

Directions:

1. Season chicken breasts with salt and pepper, put in preheated air fryer and cook at 350 degrees F for 10 minutes.

2. Meanwhile, heat up a pan with the chili sauce over medium heat, add ketchup, pear jelly, honey, liquid smoke, chili powder, mustard powder, sweet paprika, salt, pepper and the garlic powder, stir, bring to a simmer and cook for 10 minutes.
3. Add air fried chicken breasts, toss well, divide among plates and serve.

Enjoy!

Nutrition: calories 473, fat 13, fiber 7, carbs 39, protein 33

Duck Breasts And Mango Mix

Preparation time: 1 hour **Cooking time:** 10 minutes **Servings:** 4

Ingredients:

- 4 duck breasts
- 1 and ½ tablespoons lemongrass, chopped
- 3 tablespoons lemon juice
- 2 tablespoons olive oil
- Salt and black pepper to the taste
- 3 garlic cloves, minced

For the mango mix:

- 1 mango, peeled and chopped
- 1 tablespoon coriander, chopped
- 1 red onion, chopped
- 1 tablespoon sweet chili sauce
- 1 and ½ tablespoon lemon juice
- 1 teaspoon ginger, grated
- ¾ teaspoon sugar

Directions:

1. In a bowl, mix duck breasts with salt, pepper, lemongrass, 3 tablespoons lemon juice, olive oil and garlic, toss well, keep in the fridge for 1 hour, transfer to your air fryer and cook at 360 degrees F for 10 minutes, flipping once.
2. Meanwhile, in a bowl, mix mango with coriander, onion, chili sauce, lemon juice, ginger and sugar and toss well.
3. Divide duck on plates, add mango mix on the side and serve.

Enjoy!

Nutrition: calories 465, fat 11, fiber 4, carbs 29, protein 38

Quick Creamy Chicken Casserole

Preparation time: 10 minutes **Cooking time:** 12 minutes
Servings: 4

Ingredients:

- 10 ounces spinach, chopped
- 4 tablespoons butter
- 3 tablespoons flour
- 1 and ½ cups milk
- ½ cup parmesan, grated
- ½ cup heavy cream
- Salt and black pepper to the taste
- 2 cup chicken breasts, skinless, boneless and cubed
- 1 cup bread crumbs

Directions:

1. Heat up a pan with the butter over medium heat, add flour and stir well.
2. Add milk, heavy cream and parmesan, stir well, cook for 1-2 minutes more and take off heat.
3. In a pan that fits your air fryer, spread chicken and spinach.

4. Add salt and pepper and toss.

5. Add cream mix and spread, sprinkle bread crumbs on top, introduce in your air fryer and cook at 350 for 12 minutes.

6. Divide chicken and spinach mix on plates and serve.

Enjoy!

Nutrition: calories 321, fat 9, fiber 12, carbs 22, protein 17

Chicken and Peaches

Preparation time: 10 minutes **Cooking time:** 30 minutes

Servings: 6

Ingredients:

- 1 whole chicken, cut into medium pieces
- ¾ cup water
- 1/3 cup honey
- Salt and black pepper to the taste
- ¼ cup olive oil
- 4 peaches, halved

Directions:

1. Put the water in a pot, bring to a simmer over medium heat, add honey, whisk really well and leave aside.
2. Rub chicken pieces with the oil, season with salt and pepper, place in your air fryer's basket and cook at 350 degrees F for 10 minutes.
3. Brush chicken with some of the honey mix, cook for 6 minutes more, flip again, brush one more time with the honey mix and cook for 7 minutes more.
4. Divide chicken pieces on plates and keep warm.

5. Brush peaches with what's left of the honey marinade, place them in your air fryer and cook them for 3 minutes.
6. Divide among plates next to chicken pieces and serve.

Enjoy!

Nutrition: calories 430, fat 14, fiber 3, carbs 15, protein 20

Tea Glazed Chicken

Preparation time: 10 minutes **Cooking time:** 30 minutes

Servings: 6

Ingredients:

- ½ cup apricot preserves
- ½ cup pineapple preserves
- 6 chicken legs
- 1 cup hot water
- 6 black tea bags
- 1 tablespoon soy sauce
- 1 onion, chopped
- ¼ teaspoon red pepper flakes
- 1 tablespoon olive oil
- Salt and black pepper to the taste
- 6 chicken legs

Directions:

1. Put the hot water in a bowl, add tea bags, leave aside covered for 10 minutes, discard bags at the end and transfer tea to another bowl.

2. Add soy sauce, pepper flakes, apricot and pineapple preserves, whisk really well and take off heat.

3. Season chicken with salt and pepper, rub with oil, put in your air fryer and cook at 350 degrees F for 5 minutes.

4. Spread onion on the bottom of a baking dish that fits your air fryer, add chicken pieces, drizzle the tea glaze on top, introduce in your air fryer and cook at 320 degrees F for 25 minutes.

5. Divide everything on plates and serve.

Enjoy!

Nutrition: calories 298, fat 14, fiber 1, carbs 14, protein 30

Chicken and Radish Mix

Preparation time: 10 minutes **Cooking time:** 30 minutes

Servings: 4

Ingredients:

- 4 chicken things, bone-in
- Salt and black pepper to the taste
- 1 tablespoon olive oil
- 1 cup chicken stock
- 6 radishes, halved
- 1 teaspoon sugar
- 3 carrots, cut into thin sticks
- 2 tablespoon chives, chopped

Directions:

1. Heat up a pan that fits your air fryer over medium heat, add stock, carrots, sugar and radishes, stir gently, reduce heat to medium, cover pot partly and simmer for 20 minutes.
2. Rub chicken with olive oil, season with salt and pepper, put in your air fryer and cook at 350 degrees F for 4 minutes.
3. Add chicken to radish mix, toss, introduce everything in your air fryer, cook for 4 minutes more, divide among plates and serve.

Enjoy!

Nutrition: calories 237, fat 10, fiber 4, carbs 19, protein 29

Air Fryer Meat Recipes

Flavored Rib Eye Steak

Preparation time: 10 minutes **Cooking time:** 20 minutes
Servings: 4

Ingredients:

- 2 pounds rib eye steak
- Salt and black pepper to the taste
- 1 tablespoons olive oil

For the rub:

- 3 tablespoons sweet paprika
- 2 tablespoons onion powder
- 2 tablespoons garlic powder
- 1 tablespoon brown sugar
- 2 tablespoons oregano, dried
- 1 tablespoon cumin, ground
- 1 tablespoon rosemary, dried

Directions:

1. In a bowl, mix paprika with onion and garlic powder, sugar, oregano, rosemary, salt, pepper and cumin, stir and rub steak with this mix.
2. Season steak with salt and pepper, rub again with the oil, put in your air fryer and cook at 400 degrees F for 20 minutes, flipping them halfway.
3. Transfer steak to a cutting board, slice and serve with a side salad.

Enjoy!

Nutrition: calories 320, fat 8, fiber 7, carbs 22, protein 21

Chinese Steak and Broccoli

Preparation time: 45 minutes **Cooking time:** 12 minutes
Servings: 4

Ingredients:

- ¾ pound round steak, cut into strips
- 1 pound broccoli florets
- 1/3 cup oyster sauce
- 2 teaspoons sesame oil
- 1 teaspoon soy sauce
- 1 teaspoon sugar
- 1/3 cup sherry
- 1 tablespoon olive oil
- 1 garlic clove, minced

Directions:

1. In a bowl, mix sesame oil with oyster sauce, soy sauce, sherry and sugar, stir well, add beef, toss and leave aside for 30 minutes.
2. Transfer beef to a pan that fits your air fryer, also add broccoli, garlic and oil, toss everything and cook at 380 degrees F for 12 minutes.
3. Divide among plates and serve.

Enjoy!

Nutrition: calories 330, fat 12, fiber 7, carbs 23, protein 23

Provencal Pork

Preparation time: 10 minutes **Cooking time:** 15 minutes

Servings: 2

Ingredients:

- 1 red onion, sliced
- 1 yellow bell pepper, cut into strips
- 1 green bell pepper, cut into strips
- Salt and black pepper to the taste
- 2 teaspoons Provencal herbs
- ½ tablespoon mustard
- 1 tablespoon olive oil
- 7 ounces pork tenderloin

Directions:

1. In a baking dish that fits your air fryer, mix yellow bell pepper with green bell pepper, onion, salt, pepper, Provencal herbs and half of the oil and toss well.
2. Season pork with salt, pepper, mustard and the rest of the oil, toss well and add to veggies.
3. Introduce everything in your air fryer, cook at 370 degrees F for 15 minutes, divide among plates and serve.

Enjoy!

Nutrition: calories 300, fat 8, fiber 7, carbs 21, protein 23

Beef S trips with Snow Peas and Mushrooms

Preparation time: 10 minutes **Cooking time:** 22 minutes

Servings: 2

Ingredients:

- 2 beef steaks, cut into strips
- Salt and black pepper to the taste
- 7 ounces snow peas
- 8 ounces white mushrooms, halved
- 1 yellow onion, cut into rings
- 2 tablespoons soy sauce
- 1 teaspoon olive oil

Directions:

1. In a bowl, mix olive oil with soy sauce, whisk, add beef strips and toss.
2. In another bowl, mix snow peas, onion and mushrooms with salt, pepper and the oil, toss well, put in a pan that fits your air fryer and cook at 350 degrees F for 16 minutes.
3. Add beef strips to the pan as well and cook at 400 degrees F for 6 minutes more.
4. Divide everything on plates and serve.

Enjoy!

Nutrition: calories 235, fat 8, fiber 2, carbs 22, protein 24

Garlic Lamb Chops

Preparation time: 10 minutes **Cooking time:** 10 minutes

Servings: 4

Ingredients:

- 3 tablespoons olive oil
- 8 lamb chops
- Salt and black pepper to the taste
- 4 garlic cloves, minced
- 1 tablespoon oregano, chopped
- 1 tablespoon coriander, chopped

Directions:

1. In a bowl, mix oregano with salt, pepper, oil, garlic and lamb chops and toss to coat.
2. Transfer lamb chops to your air fryer and cook at 400 degrees F for 10 minutes.
3. Divide lamb chops on plates and serve with a side salad.

Enjoy!

Nutrition: calories 231, fat 7, fiber 5, carbs 14, protein 23

Crispy Lamb

Preparation time: 10 minutes **Cooking time:** 30 minutes

Servings: 4

Ingredients:

- 1 tablespoon bread crumbs
- 2 tablespoons macadamia nuts, toasted and crushed
- 1 tablespoon olive oil
- 1 garlic clove, minced
- 28 ounces rack of lamb
- Salt and black pepper to the taste
- 1 egg,
- 1 tablespoon rosemary, chopped

Directions:

1. In a bowl, mix oil with garlic and stir well.
2. Season lamb with salt, pepper and brush with the oil.
3. In another bowl, mix nuts with breadcrumbs and rosemary.
4. Put the egg in a separate bowl and whisk well.
5. Dip lamb in egg, then in macadamia mix, place them in your air fryer's basket, cook at 360 degrees F and cook for 25 minutes, increase heat to 400 degrees F and cook for 5 minutes more.
6. Divide among plates and serve right away.

Enjoy!

Nutrition: calories 230, fat 2, fiber 2, carbs 10, protein 12

Indian Pork

Preparation time: 35 minutes **Cooking time:** 10 minutes

Servings: 4

Ingredients:

- 1 teaspoon ginger powder
- 2 teaspoons chili paste
- 2 garlic cloves, minced
- 14 ounces pork chops, cubed
- 1 shallot, chopped
- 1 teaspoon coriander, ground
- 7 ounces coconut milk
- 2 tablespoons olive oil
- 3 ounces peanuts, ground
- 3 tablespoons soy sauce
- Salt and black pepper to the taste

Directions:

1. In a bowl, mix ginger with 1 teaspoon chili paste, half of the garlic, half of the soy sauce and half of the oil, whisk, add meat, toss and leave aside for 10 minutes.
2. Transfer meat to your air fryer's basket and cook at 400 degrees F for 12 minutes, turning halfway.
3. Meanwhile, heat up a pan with the rest of the oil over medium high heat, add shallot, the rest of the garlic, coriander, coconut milk, the rest of the peanuts, the rest of the chili paste and the rest of the soy sauce, stir and cook for 5 minutes.
4. Divide pork on plates, spread coconut mix on top and serve.

Enjoy!

Nutrition: calories 423, fat 11, fiber 4, carbs 42, protein 18

Lamb and Creamy Brussels Sprouts

Preparation time: 10 minutes **Cooking time:** 1 hour and 10 minutes **Servings:** 4

Ingredients:

- 2 pounds leg of lamb, scored
- 2 tablespoons olive oil
- 1 tablespoon rosemary, chopped
- 1 tablespoon lemon thyme, chopped
- 1 garlic clove, minced
- 1 and ½ pounds Brussels sprouts, trimmed
- 1 tablespoon butter, melted
- ½ cup sour cream
- Salt and black pepper to the taste

Directions:

1. Season leg of lamb with salt, pepper, thyme and rosemary, brush with oil, place in your air fryer's basket, cook at 300 degrees F for 1 hour, transfer to a plate and keep warm.
2. In a pan that fits your air fryer, mix Brussels sprouts with salt, pepper, garlic, butter and sour cream, toss, put in your air fryer and cook at 400 degrees F for 10 minutes.
3. Divide lamb on plates, add Brussels sprouts on the side and serve.

Enjoy!

Nutrition: calories 440, fat 23, fiber 0, carbs 2, protein 49

Beef Fillets with Garlic Mayo

Preparation time: 10 minutes **Cooking time:** 40 minutes
Servings: 8

Ingredients:

- 1 cup mayonnaise
- 1/3 cup sour cream
- 2 garlic cloves, minced
- 3 pounds beef fillet
- 2 tablespoons chives, chopped
- 2 tablespoons mustard
- 2 tablespoons mustard
- ¼ cup tarragon, chopped
- Salt and black pepper to the taste

Directions:

1. Season beef with salt and pepper to the taste, place in your air fryer, cook at 370 degrees F for 20 minutes, transfer to a plate and leave aside for a few minutes.
2. In a bowl, mix garlic with sour cream, chives, mayo, some salt and pepper, whisk and leave aside.

3. In another bowl, mix mustard with Dijon mustard and tarragon, whisk, add beef, toss, return to your air fryer and cook at 350 degrees F for 20 minutes more.
4. Divide beef on plates, spread garlic mayo on top and serve.

Enjoy!

Nutrition: calories 400, fat 12, fiber 2, carbs 27, protein 19

Mustard Marina ted Beef

Preparation time: 10 minutes **Cooking time:** 45 minutes

Servings: 6

Ingredients:

- 6 bacon strips
- 2 tablespoons butter
- 3 garlic cloves, minced
- Salt and black pepper to the taste
- 1 tablespoon horseradish
- 1 tablespoon mustard
- 3 pounds beef roast
- 1 and ¾ cup beef stock
- ¾ cup red wine

Directions:

1. In a bowl, mix butter with mustard, garlic, salt, pepper and horseradish, whisk and rub beef with this mix.
2. Arrange bacon strips on a cutting board, place beef on top, fold bacon around beef, transfer to your air fryer's basket, cook at 400 degrees F for 15 minutes and transfer to a pan that fits your fryer.

3. Add stock and wine to beef, introduce pan in your air fryer and cook at 360 degrees F for 30 minutes more.
4. Carve beef, divide among plates and serve with a side salad.

Enjoy!

Nutrition: calories 500, fat 9, fiber 4, carbs 29, protein 36

Creamy Pork

Preparation time: 10 minutes **Cooking time:** 22 minutes

Servings: 6

Ingredients:

- 2 pounds pork meat, boneless and cubed
- 2 yellow onions, chopped
- 1 tablespoon olive oil
- 1 garlic clove, minced
- 3 cups chicken stock
- 2 tablespoons sweet paprika
- Salt and black pepper to the taste
- 2 tablespoons white flour
- 1 and ½ cups sour cream
- 2 tablespoons dill, chopped

Directions:

1. In a pan that fits your air fryer, mix pork with salt, pepper and oil, toss, introduce in your air fryer and cook at 360 degrees F for 7 minutes.
2. Add onion, garlic, stock, paprika, flour, sour cream and dill, toss and cook at 370 degrees F for 15 minutes more.
3. Divide everything on plates and serve right away.

Enjoy!

Nutrition: calories 300, fat 4, fiber 10, carbs 26, protein 34

Marinated Pork Chops and Onions

Preparation time: 24 hours **Cooking time:** 25 minutes **Servings:** 6

Ingredients:

- 2 pork chops
- ¼ cup olive oil
- 2 yellow onions, sliced
- 2 garlic cloves, minced
- 2 teaspoons mustard
- 1 teaspoon sweet paprika
- Salt and black pepper to the taste
- ½ teaspoon oregano, dried
- ½ teaspoon thyme, dried
- A pinch of cayenne pepper

Directions:

1. In a bowl, mix oil with garlic, mustard, paprika, black pepper, oregano, thyme and cayenne and whisk well.
2. Combine onions with meat and mustard mix, toss to coat, cover and keep in the fridge for 1 day.

3. Transfer meat and onions mix to a pan that fits your air fryer and cook at 360 degrees F for 25 minutes.
4. Divide everything on plates and serve.

Enjoy!

Nutrition: calories 384, fat 4, fiber 4, carbs 17, protein 25

Simple Braised Pork

Preparation time: 40 minutes **Cooking time:** 40 minutes
Servings: 4

Ingredients:

- 2 pounds pork loin roast, boneless and cubed
- 4 tablespoons butter, melted
- Salt and black pepper to the taste
- 2 cups chicken stock
- ½ cup dry white wine
- 2 garlic cloves, minced
- 1 teaspoon thyme, chopped
- 1 thyme spring
- 1 bay leaf
- ½ yellow onion, chopped
- 2 tablespoons white flour
- ½ pound red grapes

Directions:

1. Season pork cubes with salt and pepper, rub with 2 tablespoons melted butter, put in your air fryer and cook at 370 degrees F for 8 minutes.

2. Meanwhile, heat up a pan that fits your air fryer with 2 tablespoons butter over medium high heat, add garlic and onion, stir and cook for 2 minutes.
3. Add wine, stock, salt, pepper, thyme, flour and bay leaf, stir well, bring to a simmer and take off heat.
4. Add pork cubes and grapes, toss, introduce in your air fryer and cook at 360 degrees F for 30 minutes more.
5. Divide everything on plates and serve.

Enjoy!

Nutrition: calories 320, fat 4, fiber 5, carbs 29, protein 38

Pork with Couscous

Preparation time: 10 minutes **Cooking time:** 35 minutes

Servings: 6

Ingredients:

- 2 and ½ pounds pork loin, boneless and trimmed
- ¾ cup chicken stock
- 2 tablespoons olive oil
- ½ tablespoon sweet paprika
- 2 and ¼ teaspoon sage, dried
- ½ tablespoon garlic powder
- ¼ teaspoon rosemary, dried
- ¼ teaspoon marjoram, dried
- 1 teaspoon basil, dried
- 1 teaspoon oregano, dried
- Salt and black pepper to the taste
- 2 cups couscous, cooked

Directions:

1. In a bowl, mix oil with stock, paprika, garlic powder, sage, rosemary, thyme, marjoram, oregano, salt and

pepper to the taste, whisk well, add pork loin, toss well and leave aside for 1 hour.

2. Transfer everything to a pan that fits your air fryer and cook at 370 degrees F for 35 minutes.

3. Divide among plates and serve with couscous on the side.

Enjoy!

Nutrition: calories 310, fat 4, fiber 6, carbs 37, protein 34

Simple Air Fried Pork Shoulder

Preparation time: 30 minutes **Cooking time:** 1 hour and 20 minutes **Servings:** 6

Ingredients:

- 3 tablespoons garlic, minced
- 3 tablespoons olive oil
- 4 pounds pork shoulder
- Salt and black pepper to the taste

Directions:

1. In a bowl, mix olive oil with salt, pepper and oil, whisk well and brush pork shoulder with this mix.
2. Place in preheated air fryer and cook at 390 degrees F for 10 minutes.
3. Reduce heat to 300 degrees F and roast pork for 1 hour and 10 minutes.
4. Slice pork shoulder, divide among plates and serve with a side salad.

Enjoy!

Nutrition: calories 221, fat 4, fiber 4, carbs 7, protein 10

Fennel Flavored Pork Roast

Preparation time: 10 minutes **Cooking time:** 1 hour **Servings:** 10

Ingredients:

- 5 and ½ pounds pork loin roast, trimmed
- Salt and black pepper to the taste
- 3 garlic cloves, minced
- 2 tablespoons rosemary, chopped
- 1 teaspoon fennel, ground
- 1 tablespoon fennel seeds
- 2 teaspoons red pepper, crushed
- ¼ cup olive oil

Directions:

1. In your food processor mix garlic with fennel seeds, fennel, rosemary, red pepper, some black pepper and the olive oil and blend until you obtain a paste.
2. Spread 2 tablespoons garlic paste on pork loin, rub well, season with salt and pepper, introduce in your preheated air fryer and cook at 350 degrees F for 30 minutes.
3. Reduce heat to 300 degrees F and cook for 15 minutes more.
4. Slice pork, divide among plates and serve.

Enjoy!

Nutrition: calories 300, fat 14, fiber 9, carbs 26, protein 22

Beef Brisket and Onion Sauce

Preparation time: 10 minutes **Cooking time:** 2 hours **Servings:** 6

Ingredients:

- 1 pound yellow onion, chopped
- 4 pounds beef brisket
- 1 pound carrot, chopped
- 8 earl grey tea bags
- ½ pound celery, chopped
- Salt and black pepper to the taste
- 4 cups water

For the sauce:

- 16 ounces canned tomatoes, chopped
- ½ pound celery, chopped
- 1 ounce garlic, minced
- 4 ounces vegetable oil
- 1 pound sweet onion, chopped
- 1 cup brown sugar
- 8 earl grey tea bags
- 1 cup white vinegar

Directions:

1. Put the water in a heat proof dish that fits your air fryer, add 1 pound onion, 1 pound carrot, ½ pound celery, salt and pepper, stir and bring to a simmer over medium high heat.
2. Add beef brisket and 8 tea bags, stir, transfer to your air fryer and cook at 300 degrees F for 1 hour and 30 minutes.
3. Meanwhile, heat up a pan with the vegetable oil over medium high heat, add 1 pound onion, stir and sauté for 10 minutes.
4. Add garlic, ½ pound celery, tomatoes, sugar, vinegar, salt, pepper and 8 tea bags, stir, bring to a simmer, cook for 10 minutes and discard tea bags.
5. Transfer beef brisket to a cutting board, slice, divide among plates, drizzle onion sauce all over and serve.

Enjoy!

Nutrition: calories 400, fat 12, fiber 4, carbs 38, protein 34

Beef and Green Onions Marinade

Preparation time: 10 minutes **Cooking time:** 20 minutes

Servings: 4

Ingredients:

- 1 cup green onion, chopped
- 1 cup soy sauce
- ½ cup water
- ¼ cup brown sugar
- ¼ cup sesame seeds
- 5 garlic cloves, minced
- 1 teaspoon black pepper
- 1 pound lean beef

Directions:

1. In a bowl, mix onion with soy sauce, water, sugar, garlic, sesame seeds and pepper, whisk, add meat, toss and leave aside for 10 minutes.
2. Drain beef, transfer to your preheated air fryer and cook at 390 degrees F for 20 minutes.
3. Slice, divide among plates and serve with a side salad.

Enjoy!

Nutrition: calories 329, fat 8, fiber 12, carbs 26, protein 22

Garlic and Bell Pepper Beef

Preparation time: 30 minutes **Cooking time:** 30 minutes

Servings: 4

Ingredients:

- 11 ounces steak fillets, sliced
- 4 garlic cloves, minced
- 2 tablespoons olive oil
- 1 red bell pepper, cut into strips
- Black pepper to the taste
- 1 tablespoon sugar
- 2 tablespoons fish sauce
- 2 teaspoons corn flour
- ½ cup beef stock
- 4 green onions, sliced

Directions:

1. In a pan that fits your air fryer mix beef with oil, garlic, black pepper and bell pepper, stir, cover and keep in the fridge for 30 minutes.
2. Put the pan in your preheated air fryer and cook at 360 degrees F for 14 minutes.
3. In a bowl, mix sugar with fish sauce, stir well, pour over beef and cook at 360 degrees F for 7 minutes more.
4. Add stock mixed with corn flour and green onions, toss and cook at 370 degrees F for 7 minutes more.
5. Divide everything on plates and serve.

Enjoy!

Nutrition: calories 343, fat 3, fiber 12, carbs 26, protein 38

Marinated Lamb and Veggies

Preparation time: 10 minutes **Cooking time:** 30 minutes

Servings: 4

Ingredients:

- 1 carrot, chopped
- 1 onion, sliced
- ½ tablespoon olive oil
- 3 ounces bean sprouts
- 8 ounces lamb loin, sliced

For the marinade:

- 1 garlic clove, minced
- ½ apple, grated
- Salt and black pepper to the taste
- 1 small yellow onion, grated
- 1 tablespoon ginger, grated
- 5 tablespoons soy sauce
- 1 tablespoons sugar
- 2 tablespoons orange juice

Directions:

1. In a bowl, mix 1 grated onion with the apple, garlic, 1 tablespoon ginger, soy sauce, orange juice, sugar and black pepper, whisk well, add lamb and leave aside for 10 minutes.
2. Heat up a pan that fits your air fryer with the olive oil over medium high heat, add 1 sliced onion, carrot and bean sprouts, stir and cook for 3 minutes.
3. Add lamb and the marinade, transfer pan to your preheated air fryer and cook at 360 degrees F for 25 minutes.
4. Divide everything into bowls and serve.

Enjoy!

Nutrition: calories 265, fat 3, fiber 7, carbs 18, protein 22

Creamy Lamb

Preparation time: 3 hours **Cooking time:** 1 hour **Servings:** 8

Ingredients:

- 5 pounds leg of lamb
- 2 cups low fat buttermilk
- 2 tablespoons mustard
- ½ cup butter
- 2 tablespoons basil, chopped
- 2 tablespoons tomato paste
- 2 garlic cloves, minced
- Salt and black pepper to the taste
- 1 cup white wine
- 1 tablespoon cornstarch mixed with 1 tablespoon water
- ½ cup sour cream

Directions:

1. Put lamb roast in a big dish, add buttermilk, toss to coat, cover and keep in the fridge for 24 hours.
2. Pat dry lamb and put in a pan that fits your air fryer.
3. In a bowl, mix butter with tomato paste, mustard, basil, rosemary, salt, pepper and garlic, whisk well, spread over lamb, introduce everything in your air fryer and cook at 300 degrees F for 1 hour.
4. Slice lamb, divide among plates, leave aside for now and heat up cooking juices from the pan on your stove.
5. Add wine, cornstarch mix, salt, pepper and sour cream, stir, take off heat, drizzle this sauce over lamb and serve.

Enjoy!

Nutrition: calories 287, fat 4, fiber 7, carbs 19, protein 25

Blueberry Pudding

Preparation time: 10 minutes **Cooking time:** 25 minutes

Servings: 6

Ingredients:

- 2 cups flour
- 2 cups rolled oats
- 8 cups blueberries
- 1 stick butter, melted
- 1 cup walnuts, chopped
- 3 tablespoons maple syrup
- 2 tablespoons rosemary, chopped

Directions:

1. Spread blueberries in a greased baking pan and leave aside.
2. In your food processor, mix rolled oats with flour, walnuts, butter, maple syrup and rosemary, blend well, layer this over blueberries, introduce everything in your air fryer and cook at 350 degrees for 25 minutes.
3. Leave dessert to cool down, cut and serve.
   Enjoy!

Nutrition: calories 150, fat 3, fiber 2, carbs 7, protein 4

Cocoa and Almond Bars

Preparation time: 30 minutes **Cooking time:** 4 minutes

Servings: 6

Ingredients:

- ¼ cup cocoa nibs
- 1 cup almonds, soaked and drained
- 2 tablespoons cocoa powder
- ¼ cup hemp seeds
- ¼ cup goji berries
- ¼ cup coconut, shredded
- 8 dates, pitted and soaked

Directions:

1. Put almonds in your food processor, blend, add hemp seeds, cocoa nibs, cocoa powder, goji, coconut and blend very well.

2. Add dates, blend well again, spread on a lined baking sheet that fits your air fryer and cook at 320 degrees F for 4 minutes.

3. Cut into equal parts and keep in the fridge for 30 minutes before serving.

Enjoy!

Nutrition: calories 140, fat 6, fiber 3, carbs 7, protein 19

Chocolate and Pomegranate Bars

Preparation time: 2 hours **Cooking time:** 10 minutes **Servings:** 6

Ingredients:

- ½ cup milk
- 1 teaspoon vanilla extract
- 1 and ½ cups dark chocolate, chopped
- ½ cup almonds, chopped
- ½ cup pomegranate seeds

Directions:

1. Heat up a pan with the milk over medium low heat, add chocolate, stir for 5 minutes, take off heat add vanilla extract, half of the pomegranate seeds and half of the nuts and stir.

2. Pour this into a lined baking pan, spread, sprinkle a pinch of salt, the rest of the pomegranate arils and nuts, introduce in your air fryer and cook at 300 degrees F for 4 minutes.

3. Keep in the fridge for 2 hours before serving.

Enjoy!

Nutrition: calories 68, fat 1, fiber 4, carbs 6, protein 1

Tomato Cake

Preparation time: 10 minutes **Cooking time:** 30 minutes

Servings: 4

Ingredients:

- 1 and ½ cups flour
- 1 teaspoon cinnamon powder
- 1 teaspoon baking powder
- 1 teaspoon baking soda
- ¾ cup maple syrup
- 1 cup tomatoes chopped
- ½ cup olive oil
- 2 tablespoon apple cider vinegar

Directions:

1. In a bowl, mix flour with baking powder, baking soda, cinnamon and maple syrup and stir well.
2. In another bowl, mix tomatoes with olive oil and vinegar and stir well.
3. Combine the 2 mixtures, stir well, pour into a greased round pan that fits your air fryer, introduce in the fryer and cook at 360 degrees F for 30 minutes.
4. Leave cake to cool down, slice and serve.

Enjoy!

Nutrition: calories 153, fat 2, fiber 1, carbs 25, protein 4

Berries Mix

Preparation time: 5 minutes **Cooking time:** 6 minutes **Servings:** 4

Ingredients:

- 2 tablespoons lemon juice
- 1 and ½ tablespoons maple syrup
- 1 and ½ tablespoons champagne vinegar
- 1 tablespoon olive oil
- 1 pound strawberries, halved
- 1 and ½ cups blueberries
- ¼ cup basil leaves, torn

Directions:

1. In a pan that fits your air fryer, mix lemon juice with maple syrup and vinegar, bring to a boil over medium high heat, add oil, blueberries and strawberries, stir, introduce in your air fryer and cook at 310 degrees F for 6 minutes.
2. Sprinkle basil on top and serve!

Enjoy!

Lemon Tart

Preparation time: 1 hour **Cooking time:** 35 minutes **Servings:** 6

Ingredients:

For the crust:

- 2 tablespoons sugar
- 2 cups white flour
- A pinch of salt
- 3 tablespoons ice water
- 12 tablespoons cold butter

For the filling:

- 2 eggs, whisked
- 1 and ¼ cup sugar
- 10 tablespoons melted and chilled butter
- Juice from 2 lemons
- Zest from 2 lemons, grated

Directions:

1. In a bowl, mix 2 cups flour with a pinch of salt and 2 tablespoons sugar and whisk.
2. Add 12 tablespoons butter and the water, knead until you obtain a dough, shape a ball, wrap in foil and keep in the fridge for 1 hour.
3. Transfer dough to a floured surface, flatten it, arrange on the bottom of a tart pan, prick with a fork, keep in the fridge for 20 minutes, introduce in your air fryer at 360 degrees F and bake for 15 minutes.
4. In a bowl, mix 1 and ¼ cup sugar with eggs, 10 tablespoons butter, lemon juice and lemon zest and whisk very well.
5. Pour this into pie crust, spread evenly, introduce in the fryer and cook at 360 degrees F for 20 minutes.
6. Cut and serve it.

Enjoy!

Nutrition: calories 182, fat 4, fiber 1, carbs 2, protein 3

Mandarin Pudding

Preparation time: 20 minutes **Cooking time:** 40 minutes
Servings: 8

Ingredients:

- 1 mandarin, peeled and sliced
- Juice from 2 mandarins
- 2 tablespoons brown sugar
- 4 ounces butter, soft
- 2 eggs, whisked
- ¾ cup sugar
- ¾ cup white flour
- ¾ cup almonds, ground
- Honey for serving

Directions:

1. Grease a loaf pan with some butter, sprinkle brown sugar on the bottom and arrange mandarin slices.
2. In a bowl, mix butter with sugar, eggs, almonds, flour and mandarin juice, stir, spoon this over mandarin slices, place pan in your air fryer and cook at 360 degrees F for 40 minutes.
3. Transfer pudding to a plate and serve with honey on top.

Enjoy!

Nutrition: calories 162, fat 3, fiber 2, carbs 3, protein 6

Strawberry Shortcakes

Preparation time: 20 minutes **Cooking time:** 45 minutes

Servings: 6

Ingredients:

- Cooking spray
- ¼ cup sugar+ 4 tablespoons
- 1 and ½ cup flour
- 1 teaspoon baking powder
- ¼ teaspoon baking soda
- 1/3 cup butter
- 1 cup buttermilk
- 1 egg, whisked
- 2 cups strawberries, sliced
- 1 tablespoon rum
- 1 tablespoon mint, chopped
- 1 teaspoon lime zest, grated
- ½ cup whipping cream

Directions:

1. In a bowl, mix flour with ¼ cup sugar, baking powder and baking soda and stir.
2. In another bowl, mix buttermilk with egg, stir, add to flour mix and whisk.
3. Spoon this dough into 6 jars greased with cooking spray, cover with tin foil, arrange them in your air fryer cook at 360 degrees F for 45 minutes.
4. Meanwhile, in a bowl, mix strawberries with 3 tablespoons sugar, rum, mint and lime zest, stir and leave aside in a cold place.
5. In another bowl, mix whipping cream with 1 tablespoon sugar and stir.
6. Take jars out, divide strawberry mix and whipped cream on top and serve.

Enjoy!

Nutrition: calories 164, fat 2, fiber 3, carbs 5, protein 2

CPSIA information can be obtained
at www.ICGtesting.com
Printed in the USA
BVHW061850050421
604208BV00002B/457

MW01230889

Daily Keto Living

Meat, Fish, Soups, Vegetables & Extra Treats
Collected in a Step-by-Step Recipe Book

Kimberly Wood

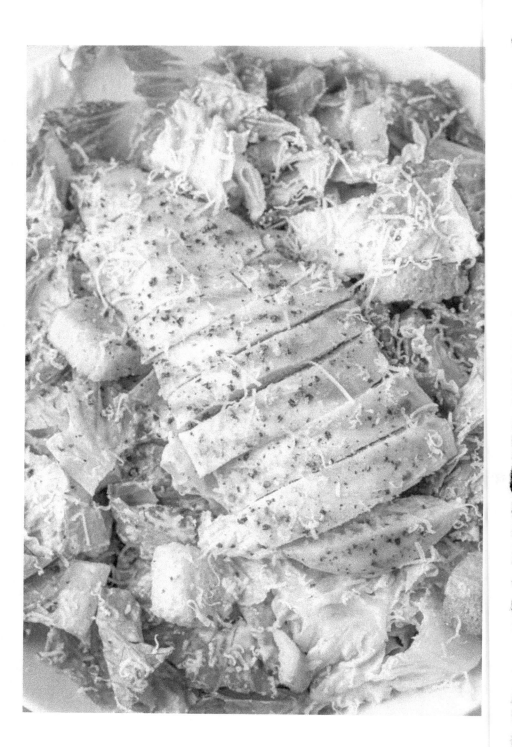

Table of Contents

POULTRY

Keto Fried Chicken With Broccoli

Marcos: Fat 85% | Protein 12% | Carbs 3%

Prep time: 5 minutes | Cook time: 15 minutes | Serves 3

Not many things could be done in 20 minutes, right? Well, you might want to reconsider that opinion because this luscious dish of broccoli and fried chicken takes only 20 minutes to prepare. I remember the first time I made this dish. It tastes like something that I would order from a Chinese restaurant but even better. It saves me through many days when I was busy, and it's delicious at the same time, so what are you waiting for? Prepare the ingredients and get yourself ready for an enjoyable journey.

- 9 ounces (255 g) broccoli
- 3½ ounces (99 g) butter
- 10ounces (284 g) boneless chicken thighs
- Salt and freshly ground black pepper, to taste
- ½ cup keto-friendly mayonnaise

Wash and cut the broccoli and the stem into small pieces.

Heat up a good amount of butter in a big frying pan where you will be able to fit both the broccoli and the chicken.

Season the chicken with salt and pepper, then fry over medium heat for 5 minutes on each side, or until it turns golden brown and cooked through. You can check by using a cooking thermometer in the thickest part, it gets fully cooked when it reaches 180°F (82°C)

Add a bit more butter and place the broccoli in the frying pan, and fry for another 2 minutes.

Season to taste with salt and pepper, and pour the remained butter on top, then serve.

STORAGE: place the leftovers in an air tight container and put it in the fridge. It lasts up to 3 days in the fridge. It lasts for about 1 month in the freezer in a freezer-safe container.

REHEAT: You could reheat it in the microwave with no problem, or in the oven at 350 □ (180 □) for 15 minutes.

SERVE IT WITH: You could serve it with a keto salad of your choice such as the grilled vegetable salad with pesto.

PER SERVING

calories: 653 | fat: 61.7g | total carbs: 6.2g | fiber: 2.3g | protein: 19.5g

Roasted Chicken Thighs And Cauliflower Puree

Marcos: Fat 70% | Protein 25% | Carbs 4%

Prep time: 3 hours 15 minutes | Cook time: 35 minutes | Serves 6

Since I'm attempting to constrain the number of carbs, I eat around evening time, I got a couple of cauliflower heads and transformed them into the smoothest, the richest purée which was the ideal backup to the succulent, flavorful chicken. What's more, the garlic! Gracious, the garlic. You folks, I could most likely live off broiled garlic. I made them alongside the chicken. At the point when cooked, the garlic turns out to be sweet and subtle, and draining them out of their papery skins is genuinely the best time you can have with your pants on.

CHICKEN THIGHS:

- 3 pounds (1.4 kg) chicken thighs, 2 thighs per serving, skin on and bone in
- 4 tablespoons olive oil
- 4 tablespoons lemon juice
- 2 tablespoons red wine vinegar
- 3 tablespoons finely cut fresh oregano
- 2 tablespoons finely cut fresh thyme
- 2 garlic diced cloves
- 2 teaspoons salt
- 1 teaspoon black pepper

CAULIFLOWER PUREE:

- 1 pound (454 g) cauliflower, cut into florets
- 3 ounces (85 g) Parmesan cheese, grated
- 3 tablespoons melted butter, unsalted
- ½ lemon, zest and juice
- 1 tablespoon olive oil

CHICKEN THIGHS:

Put the olive oil, lemon juice, red wine vinegar, oregano, thyme, diced garlic cloves, salt, and pepper in bowl or a large zip lock bag, then add the thighs and flip it on sides in the mixture to fully coat.

Seal or cover, and put in the fridge for 3 hours. Keep turning them every now and then for a better taste.

Heat the oven in advance to 400°F (205°C). Place one large baking tray, or two regular ones with parchment paper.

Take out the chicken thighs from the mixture, and gently put them skin- side up, on top of the tray(s).

Keep them in the oven for about 30 to 35 minutes, or use a cooking thermometer, and make sure that the internal temperature is 165°F (74°C), and that the skin color is golden brown. After that let it rest for 10 minutes before you serve it with the cauliflower mash.

CAULIFLOWER MASH:

Boil a pot of slightly salted on high heat, then add on the cauliflower to   the pot and boil for 2 to 5 minutes, or until tender but remain firm. Strain all the cauliflower florets in a colander, and get rid of the water.

Put the cauliflower in a food processor, along with the cheese, butter, lemon zest and juice, and olive oil. Keep pulsing until they gain a creamy and smooth consistency. You have the choice of using an immersion blender.

Salt and pepper to taste. You could put more butter or olive oil if you wish.

STORAGE: The purée could be prepared in advance and kept in the refrigerator for up to 3 days. It lasts for a month in the freezer, but make sure to keep it in a freezer-safe container. The chicken will remain for 3 to 4 days in the refrigerator in an airtight container.

REHEAT: In order to warm it up, you can place it on a dry skillet over medium heat until it gets warm enough.

SERVE IT WITH: It can be served with any keto salad of your choice. I recommend the classic Greek salad for a kind of variation.

PER SERVING

calories: 725 | fat: 57.1g | total carbs: 9.1g | fiber: 2.4g | protein: 43.5g

Delicious Fried Chicken With Broccoli

Marcos: Fat 72% | Protein 22% | Carbs 6%

Prep time: 10 minutes | Cook time: 25 minutes | Serves 4

There are too many recipes that could be done with chicken thighs, and for that every time I try a new one. Sometimes they are yummy sometimes not, so let me say this clearly. This fried thigh with broccoli and butter is one of the best recipes that I have discovered. If you are looking for a simple, basic, and flavorful approach to cook chicken. You have discovered it! These chicken thighs with broccoli and butter have become a regular in my household since they are so exquisite.

- 5 ounces (142 g) separated butter
- 1½ pounds (680 g) chicken thighs, boneless
- Salt and freshly ground black pepper, to taste
- 1 pound (454 g) broccoli
- ½ leek
- 1 tablespoon garlic, powder

Put half of the butter over medium high heat in a large frying pan to melt it.

Add salt and pepper to the chicken for seasoning, and then place it on pan. Keep flipping the chicken for 20 to 25 minutes (depends on the thighs size) until it turns brown on both of the sides, then remove them it from the pan, but keep it warm by covering it with aluminum foil or in the oven on over low heat.

While the thighs are in the oven, wash the broccoli including the stem and trim it. Slice it into small pieces. Rinse and wash the leek, but be careful to remove any sandy deposits between the layers. chop the leek into big pieces.

In a different skillet, melt the rest of the butter on medium heat, then add in the salt and pepper, and the garlic powder. Put the leek to them, and start stirring slowly until it starts to get softer, then put the broccoli. Cook it for about 5 minutes, until it becomes tender.

Serve the vegetables and chicken with an extra amount melted butter on top.

STORAGE: The chicken thighs could be stored in the refrigerator and will last for up to 4 days in the, and for 2 months in the freezer, but make sure you keep it in freezer-safe container.

REHEAT: It heats perfectly in the microwave, but you can also heat it in the oven. Heat your oven in advance to 350°F (180°C). Place the chicken wings on a baking sheet in a single layer. Put the wings in the preheated oven for about 15 to 20 minutes.

SERVE IT WITH: It could be served with keto salads of your choice such as the classic Greek salad.

PER SERVING

calories: 602 | fat: 48.3g | total carbs: 10.3g | fiber: 3.2g | protein: 32.8g

Rotisserie Chicken And Keto Chili-Flavored Béarnaise Sauce

Marcos: Fat 69% | Protein 30% | Carbs 1%

Prep time: 10 minutes | Cook time: 15 minutes | Serves 6

To Rotisserie or not to Rotisserie, that is the question! Well, it's definitely one of the most delicious dishes to me. I have tried Rotisserie chicken in many places, but it never tastes as good as the homemade one. I realized that I don't need a cook to make me Rotisserie chicken because the world's best Rotisserie chicken could come out of your own kitchen. What do you need in order to make that happen? All you need is chicken, few spices, an oven, and love.

- 2 rotisserie chickens
- 4 egg yolks
- 2 tablespoons white wine vinegar
- ½ tablespoon onion powder
- 1 finely chopped and deseeded red chili pepper
- 10 ounces (284 g) butter
- Salt and freshly ground black pepper, to taste
- 3 ounces (85 g) leafy vegetables

Split the chicken into two pieces, and make a fresh leafy salad or basically another side dish of your choice.

Crack the eggs and take only egg yolks, then put them into a heat- resistant bowl. Mix the wine vinegar, chili and onion powder in a mug, then put the butter in a saucepan and melt it.

Slowly beat the egg yolks and add the butter one drop at a time into the yolk while whisking. Increase the pace as the sauce thickens. Continue to whisk until you are done with all the butter. You'll see that white milk protein has accumulated at the pan's bottom; however, it should be removed.

Put the vinegar in, then stir together with salt and pepper to add taste.

Make sure to keep the sauce warm.

Serve it with green salad and a fried chicken or any other side dish of your choice, personally I prefer the green salad because it adds variation to the taste.

STORAGE: It lasts for up to 4 days in the refrigerator, and for 2 months in the freezer, but make sure you keep it in freezer-safe container.

REHEAT:To heat Rotisserie chicken you'll need to place it in an oven-safe dish, and roast in the oven for 25 minutes at 350°F (180°C).

SERVE IT WITH: You can serve it with any kind of green salad, two of my favorites are caprese zoodles and classic Greek salad.

PER SERVING

calories: 505 | fat: 38.9g | total carbs: 2.1g | fiber: 0.4g | protein: 37.5g

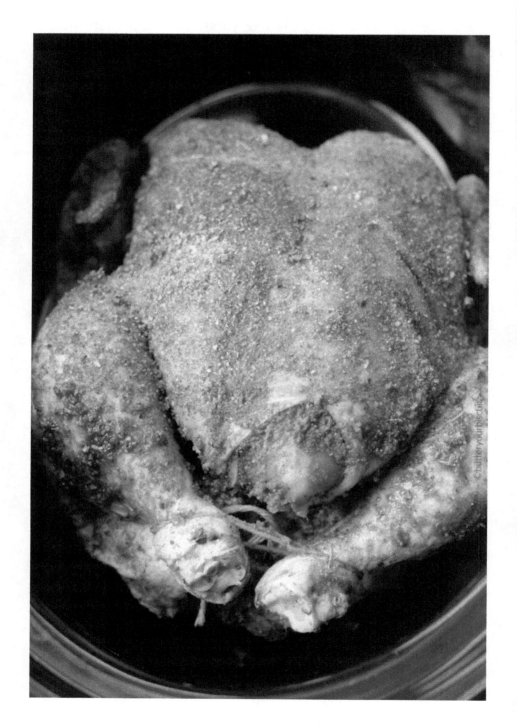

Chicken Wings And Blue Cheese Dip

Macros: Fat 58% | Protein 39%| Carbs 3%

Prep time: 1 hour | Cook time: 25 minutes | Serves 4

Something I learned in my early ages is that you simply cannot enjoy chicken wings without the blue cheese dressing. To me it feels like a rule that should be taught in school, and the equation should be that chicken wings plus blue cheese dip equals happiness. If you have never tried the blue cheese dip with chicken wings then what are you waiting for? Let your tongue enjoy the creaminess of the cheese with the mouth-watering wings.

You could have any other dip of your choice such as the curry sauce or the traditional hot sauce.

- ⅓ cup mayonnaise, keto-friendly
- ¼ cup sour cream
- 3 tablespoons lemon juice
- ¼ tablespoon garlic powder
- ¼ tablespoon salt
- ¼ cup heavy whipping cream
- 3 ounces (85 g) blue cheese, crumbled
- 2 pounds (907 g) chicken wings
- 2 tablespoons olive oil
- ¼ tablespoon garlic powder
- 1 garlic clove, minced
- 1teaspoon salt
- ¼ tablespoon ground black pepper
- 2 ounces (57 g) Parmesan cheese, grated

Put the mayonnaise, sour cream, lemon juice, garlic powder, salt, and cream in a large bowl, and whisk to combine. Add the blue cheese crumbles in and mix well.

Let it chill for about 45 minutes before you serve it. You can use this dressing over salads or as I recommend as a dip for the wings or vegetables.

Prepare the chicken wings: place the wings in large bowl. Add the olive oil, garlic powder, minced garlic, salt, and black pepper. Start stirring slowly in order to coat the chicken. Let it marinate in the fridge for 30 minutes.

Preheat the oven to 425°F (220°C).

Grill or bake in the preheated oven for about 25 minutes, or until brown and tender; the skin should be crispy.

Carefully take out the wings and place them in a large bowl, then add the Parmesan cheese. Finally, put the wings in the cheese until they are coated, and Serve warm.

REHEAT: Preheat your oven to 350°F (180°C). Place the chicken wings on a baking sheet in a single layer. Put the wings in the preheated oven for about 15 to 20 minutes.

STORAGE: The chicken wings could last for four days in the refrigerator, and make sure that you wrap the cheese dip in parchment or wax paper and keep it in the refrigerator because otherwise it won't last for more than 2 days.

SERVE IT WITH: You could add your own choice of vegetables to go along with the wings. Or you can serve it with sliced cucumber or celery.

PER SERVING

calories: 658 | fat: 42.8g | total carbs: 6.0g | fiber: 0.3g | protein: 59.6g

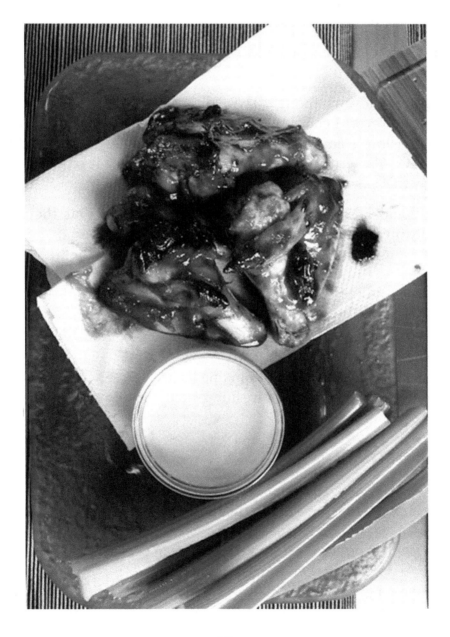

Caesar Salad

Prep time: 15 minutes | Cook time: 20 minutes | Serves 4
Marcos: Fat 78% | Protein 20% | Carbs 2%

I owe my uncle a lot since he was the one that introduced me to Caesar salad.

As a kid I always thought that salads were never meant to be tasty; however, I could recall the first time I tasted Caesar salad and the way I enjoyed it. The rich, and wonderful taste of the anchovy. The crustiness on each bite that makes it so exquisite. Enjoy this easy to make meal.

You could add edible flowers or even croutons, but they are totally optional

- ¾ pound (340 g) chicken breasts
- 1 tablespoon olive oil
- Salt and freshly ground black pepper, to taste
- 3ounces (85 g) bacon
- 7 ounces (198 g) Romaine lettuce
- 1 ounce (28 g) of freshly grated Parmesan cheese

DRESSING:

- ½ cup mayonnaise, keto-friendly
- 1 tablespoon Dijon mustard
- ½ lemon, juice and zest
- ½ ounce (14 g) grated Parmesan cheese, finely grated
- 2 tablespoons anchovy paste
- 1 garlic clove, finely chopped or pressed
- Salt and freshly ground black pepper, to taste

20

Preheat the oven to 350°F (180°C).

Spread the chicken breasts in a greased baking dish.

Add salt and pepper to the chicken, then drizzle melted butter or olive oil on top of it.

Bake the chicken in the preheated oven for 20 minutes, or until you notice that it's fully cooked through by sticking a knife into the thickest part, and making sure that the juices are colorless and smooth. (You can also check by using a cooking thermometer in the thick part, its fully cooked when it reaches 180°F (82°C)). you could also cook the chicken by using the stovetop.

Fry the bacon until it gets crispy. Chop the lettuce and put it as a base on two plates, then place the crispy, crumbles bacon on top of the sliced pieces of chicken.

In order to make the dressing, put the ingredients in a bowl and mix them with a whisk or with an immersion blender, then set it aside in the refrigerator.

End it with a good dollop of dressing and a fine grating of the cheese.

STORAGE: It lasts for about 3 to 5 days in the refrigerator, but it might lose the crispiness on the second day.

REHEAT: You could heat the cold left-over sliced chicken pieces by frying them in a small amount of butter for a delicious, warm addition.

SERVE IT WITH: If you want to serve it side by side with something, then you can make the salad basically go with any type of meat of your choice.

PER SERVING

calories: 521 | fat: 44.5g | total carbs: 4.4g | fiber: 1.3g | protein: 26.0g

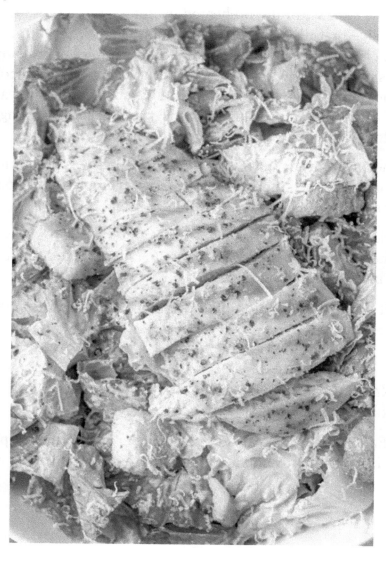

Chicken Provençale

Marcos: Fat 77% | Protein 20% | Carbs 3%

Prep time: 10 minutes | Cook time: 45 minutes | Serves 6 to 8

Do you want to have a quick trip to France in the middle of a busy week? Then you must try this chicken Provençale. I tried it the first time when I travelled to France for a week with my family, and ever since then, this meal has a special place in my heart for its unique flavor that I don't get to taste in everyday meals. The perfect balance between the ingredients in this dish takes it to a whole different level from every day to day meals, so treat yourself with an exquisite meal.

- 2 pounds (907 g) chicken drumsticks
- 8 ounces (227 g) tomatoes
- 2½ ounces (71 g) pitted black olives
- ¼ cup olive oil
- 5 sliced garlic cloves
- 1 tablespoon dried oregano
- Salt and freshly ground black pepper, to taste

FOR SERVING:

- 7 ounces (198 g) lettuce
- 1 cup mayonnaise, keto-friendly
- ¼ lemon zest
- 1 tablespoon paprika powder
- Salt and freshly ground black pepper, to taste

Start by preheating the oven to 400°F (205°C). Set the chicken's skin side up in an oven-safe baking dish. Add olives, garlic and tomatoes on top of the meat and around it.

Drizzle over it a good amount of olive oil, then spatter it with oregano and put salt and pepper to season.

Put in the oven and roast. It should take about 45 to 60 minutes, depending on the size of the pieces. You can check internal temperature with a meat thermometer. When the temperature reaches 180°F (82°C), the chicken is cooked through. However, you could check by sticking a knife into the thickest part of the chicken, and making sure that the juices run clear.

Serve it with a salad of your choice, mayo, lemon zest, and paprika or a mild chili and a sprinkle of salt and pepper.

STORAGE: It could last for up to 4 days in a refrigerator. Allow it to cool first then wrap very well, and make sure it's away from any raw meat. It stays in the freezer for a good 2 months.

REHEAT: It could be reheated in the oven at 350°F (180°C) for about 20 minutes, and make sure you keep stirring occasionally, or by using the microwave for about 5 minutes at medium-high.

SERVE IT WITH: It could be served with salads such as the classic Greek salad or any type of keto salads of your choice.

PER SERVING

calories: 606 | fat: 51.8g | total carbs: 5.7g | fiber: 2.1g | protein: 29.0g

Chicken Breast Wrapped With Bacon And Cauliflower Purée

Macros: Fat 73% | Protein 22% | Carbs 5%

Prep time: 10 minutes | Cook time: 30 minutes | Serves 4

Have you ever thought of a meal so fancy yet so easy to make? Well, you've arrived to your destination. This bacon-wrapped chicken breast is one of my favorite meals to make, everything about it is convenient. It pretty much takes no effort to make, and exquisite at the same time. I grew up in a household full of different people with different tastes, yet they almost never refused to eat the mouth-watering bacon-wrapped chicken.

CAULIFLOWER PURÉE:

- 4 garlic cloves
- 2 ounces (57 g) butter
- ¾ pound (340 g) cauliflower
- ⅓ cup heavy whipping cream
- Salt and freshly ground black pepper, to taste

CHICKEN BREAST:

- 1 pound (454 g) chicken breast
- 10 ounces (284 g) bacon
- 2 tablespoons olive oil
- Salt and freshly ground black pepper, to taste
- 1 pound (454 g) fresh spinach

Slightly mash the garlic cloves by pressing hard on them with the handle of a knife, then peel the skin off. Fry them with butter over medium heat until they turn golden. Be careful because it can go from golden to burned in a blink of an eye, and you certainly don't want a bitter taste in your food. Turn off the heat and keep the garlic in the pan while you do the rest.

Rinse then trim the cauliflower and divide to smaller florets. Start cooking them in lightly salted water until they are tender, then remove the florets with a strainer and keep some of the water.

Place the cauliflower in a food processor or in a blender. Add garlic   cloves and the pan juices. The pan juices will add tasty flavor!

Add the cream and the purée until it turns smooth. If you wanted it thinner you could add a little bit of the reserved water to the purée. Begin with a couple of tablespoons of reserved water and keep adding more if needed, until it becomes as you desired. Season with salt and pepper to taste.

Wrap each chicken breast with one or two pieces of bacon. Put them gently in a pan and fry with olive oil until the bacon is crisp and chicken is cooked through. Keep the pan over low temperature or you could cook them in a hot oven (400°F / 205°C) for 15 minutes until an instant read thermometer inserted in the center of the chicken registers at least 165°F (74°C).

Take the chicken off the pan and keep it warm. Use the same pan to fry   the spinach, then Serve immediately with the purée.

STORAGE: The purée could be prepared ahead and stored in the refrigerator for 3 days. However, It lasts up to a month in the freezer, but be sure to keep it in a freezer-safe container.

REHEAT: In order to reheat it you can place it on a dry skillet over medium heat until it gets warm enough.

SERVE IT WITH: You can serve it with salads such as Keto Broccoli salad, or Parmesan Brussels Sprouts Salad.

PER SERVING

calories: 700 | fat: 57.3g | total carbs: 10.3g | fiber: 4.3g | protein: 38.3g

MEAT

Zesty Lamb Leg

Macros: Fat 35% | Protein 64% | Carbs 1%

Prep time: 20 minutes | Cook time: 3 hours | Serves 10

A roasted lamb leg tastes even better when it is cooked with an herb and zesty filling. In this recipe, the lamb leg is infused with all the spices like mustard, cardamom, and marjoram, and its slits are stuffed with lemon peel to give it better taste and aroma.

- 1 teaspoon salt
- 1 teaspoon seasoned salt
- ½ teaspoon black pepper
- ¼ teaspoon dry mustard
- ⅛ teaspoon ground cardamom
- ½ teaspoon dried marjoram
- 5 pounds (2.3 kg) leg of lamb
- 1 lemon peel, cut into slivers
- ½ teaspoon dried thyme Fresh mint, optional

Preheat the oven to 325 □ (160 □).

Add salt, seasoned salt, black pepper, mustard, cardamom, and marjoram in a bowl.

Mix well and rub the mixture over the lamb liberally. Cut 16 deep slits in this seasoned lamb roast with a sharp knife.

Mix lemon peel and thyme in a separate bowl and insert this dry mixture into the slits.

Place the prepared lamb roast in a roasting pan, fat-side up. Roast the lamb roast for 3 hours in the prepared oven until its internal temperature reaches 180 □ (82 □) on a meat thermometer.

Remove from the oven to a plate and garnish with fresh mint, if desired.

STORAGE: Store in a sealed airtight container in the fridge for up to 5 days or in your freezer for about 1 month.

REHEAT: Microwave, covered, until the desired temperature is reached or reheat in a frying pan or air fryer / instant pot, covered, on medium.

SERVE IT WITH: To add more flavors to this meal, serve the lamb leg on top of cauliflower rice. It also tastes great paired with sautéed Brussels sprouts.

PER SERVING

calories: 306 | fat: 12.0g | net carbs: 0.4g | fiber: 0.2g | protein: 45.9g

Wine Braised Lamb Shanks

Macros: Fat 65% | Protein 29% | Carbs 5%

Prep time: 10 minutes | Cook time: 2 hours 20 minutes | Serves 4

These wine braised lamb shanks are a simple way to make your ketogenic menu more interesting. The lamb shanks are first seared and then cooked well in a garlicky wine sauce, which gives them a unique flavor and hearty aroma. Use fresh herbs to garnish the shanks, and it will taste even better.

- 3 tablespoons olive oil
- 4 lamb shanks
- 5 garlic cloves, sliced
- 1small onion, chopped
- Salt and freshly ground black pepper, to taste
- 1 cup dry white wine
- 2 teaspoons fresh rosemary, chopped
- Rosemary sprigs, for garnish

Heat the olive oil in a large frying pan over medium-high heat.

Add lamb shanks to the hot pan, then sear them for 6 minutes per side.

Transfer the seared shanks to a plate.

Add garlic to the same pan and sauté for 30 seconds over medium-low heat.

Toss in onion and cook for about 5 minutes until soft and translucent.

Return the seared shanks to the pan.

Add salt, black pepper, rosemary, and wine. Mix well and cook covered on low heat for 2 hours, stirring occasionally. Add water if needed.

Garnish with rosemary sprigs and serve warm.

STORAGE: Store in a sealed airtight container in the fridge for up to 3 days or in your freezer for about 1 month.

REHEAT: Microwave, covered, until the desired temperature is reached or reheat in a frying pan or air fryer / instant pot, covered, on medium.

SERVE IT WITH: To add more flavors to this meal, serve the lamb shanks with tomato-cucumber salad. It also tastes great paired with cauliflower mash on the side.

PER SERVING

calories: 361 | fat: 23.3g | total carbs: 4.3g | fiber: 0.5g | protein: 23.6g

Herbed Lamb Leg

Macros: Fat 67% | Protein 33% | Carbs 0%

Prep time: 5 minutes | Cook time: 2 hours | Serves 10

Have you tried a lamb leg roasted busting with a peculiar garlicky aroma and soothing herb's flavors? Well, this recipe will offer you all of this. By using these basic ingredients, you can add a perfect balance of flavors to your lamb leg while roasting.

- 1 (5-pound / 2.3-kg) leg of lamb
- 3 garlic cloves, cut into slivers
- 1 teaspoon dried rosemary, crushed
- 1½ teaspoons salt
- 3 teaspoons dried dill weed
- ½ teaspoon ground black pepper

Preheat the oven to 325 ☐ (160 ☐).

Using a sharp knife to make a few holes in the lamb leg and stuff them with garlic slivers.

Thoroughly mix rosemary, salt, black pepper and dill in a small bowl and rub the mixture over the lamb.

Place the prepared and seasoned lamb in a roasting pan.

Roast the lamb uncovered for about 2 hours in the preheated oven. Then cover it with aluminum foil. Leave the loosely wrapped lamb for 20 minutes at room temperature.

Let cool for 8 minutes before slicing to serve.

STORAGE: Store in a sealed airtight container in the fridge for up to 5 days or in your freezer for about 1 month.

REHEAT: Microwave, covered, until the desired temperature is reached or reheat in a frying pan or air fryer / instant pot, covered, on medium.

SERVE IT WITH: To add more flavors to this meal, serve the lamb leg with cauliflower rice. It also tastes great paired with roasted broccoli florets.

PER SERVING

calories: 524 | fat: 38.8g | total carbs: 0.6g | fiber: 0.1g | protein: 40.8g

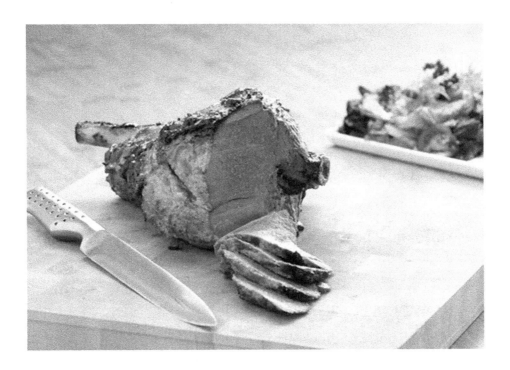

Mint Oil Braised Lamb Chops

Macros: Fat 63% | Protein 25% | Carbs 12%

Prep time: 20 minutes | Cook time: 10 minutes | Serves 4

The classic minty flavor is here to make your day. These lamb chops offer you a rich combination of healthy ingredients. The chops are cooked with basic seasoning and herbs, then it is served with special mint oil, which gives it a refreshing mint aroma and unique taste.

- 8 lamb chops
- 2 tablespoons olive oil, divided
- Salt and freshly ground black pepper, to taste
- 2 teaspoons fresh rosemary, chopped

MINT OIL:

- ¼ cup mint leaves
- 2 tablespoons extra-virgin olive oil
- 1 teaspoon lemon zest
- 1 tablespoon lemon juice

Place the lamb chops in a shallow tray and rub them evenly with 1 tablespoon olive oil, black pepper, salt, and rosemary.

Cover the seasoned lamb chops with a plastic sheet and refrigerate them for 20 minutes to 2 hours to marinate.

Heat 1 tablespoon of olive oil over medium heat.

Place the rosemary lamb chops in the skillet and sear them for 3 minutes per side until the internal temperature reaches 145°F (63°C).

Pulse mint leaves with olive oil, lemon zest, and lemon juice in a food processor until smooth.

Drizzle the mint mixture over the seared chops on a plate and serve warm.

STORAGE: Store in a sealed airtight container in the fridge for up to 3 days or in your freezer for about 1 month.

REHEAT: Microwave, covered, until the desired temperature is reached or reheat in a frying pan or air fryer / instant pot, covered, on medium.

SERVE IT WITH: To add more flavors to this meal, serve the lamb chops with cauliflower mash. It also tastes great paired with guacamole on the side.

PER SERVING

calories:278 | fat: 19.3g | total carbs: 14.0g | fiber: 5.1g | protein: 17.1g

Roasted Vietnamese Lamb Chops

Macros: Fat 57% | Protein 39% | Carbs 4%

Prep time: 10 minutes | Cook time: 25 minutes | Serves 3

If you haven't yet tried the Vietnamese lamb chops, then here is your chance to try them at home. All you need to make this delicious meal is a mixture of some spices and citrus juices to season the lamb loin chops. Then enjoy them with a hearty salad on the side.

- 5 (3-ounce / 85-g) lamb loin chops (1-inch thick)
- 1 teaspoon garlic powder, or to taste
- 2 garlic cloves, sliced
- ½ teaspoon liquid stevia
- 1 pinch chili powder
- Freshly ground black pepper, to taste
- 1 tablespoon coconut aminos
- 2 tablespoons olive oil
- 1 tablespoon fresh lime juice
- ¼ cup fresh cilantro, chopped
- 2 lime wedges
- 2 lemon wedges

Set the lamb chops in a roasting pan and combine with garlic powder, garlic, stevia, chili powder, black pepper, salt, and pepper.

Evenly sprinkle coconut aminos, olive oil, and 1 tablespoon of lime juice over the chops. Cover them with a plastic sheet and refrigerate overnight to marinate.

Preheat the oven to 400°F (205°C) and leave the lamb chops at room temperature for 10 minutes.

Uncover these chops and roast them for 25 minutes in the preheated oven.

Serve with cilantro, lemon and lime juice on top.

STORAGE: Store in a sealed airtight container in the fridge for up to 3 days or in your freezer for about 1 month.

REHEAT: Microwave, covered, until the desired temperature is reached or reheat in a frying pan or air fryer / instant pot, covered, on medium.

SERVE IT WITH: To add more flavors to this meal, serve the lamb chops with salad greens. It also tastes great paired with sautéed asparagus sticks.

PER SERVING

calories: 299 | fat: 18.9g | total carbs: 3.7g | fiber: 0.4g | protein: 28.8g

Cheesy Lamb Sliders

Macros: Fat 59% | Protein 34% | Carbs 7%

Prep time: 10 minutes | Cook time: 25 minutes | Serves 4

The dish of lamb sliders provides an interesting way to make your menu healthy and delicious. Cook the sliders with spices and serve with a feta cheese dressing. You can either serve them on top of lettuce leaves.

- 1 pound (454 g) ground lamb
- ½ teaspoon sea salt
- ½ teaspoon ground black pepper
- 2 garlic cloves, minced
- 2 teaspoons fresh oregano, leaves only
- 1 lemon, zested
- ¼ yellow onion, finely diced
- 1 tablespoon olive oil

FETA CHEESE DRESSING:

- 2 ounces (57 g) feta cheese
- ¼ cup plain Greek yogurt
- 1 garlic clove, pressed
- Salt and ground black pepper, to taste

SERVING:

- 4 lettuce leaves

- 1 tomato, sliced
- ½ red onion, sliced into rings

Preheat the grill to medium-high heat.

In a medium mixing bowl, and add ground lamb, salt, black pepper, minced garlic, oregano, lemon zest, and diced onion.

Thoroughly mix these ingredients together and keep it aside.

Make about 6 small sized lamb meat patties out of this mixture and keep them on a plate.

Lightly grease the grill grates with olive oil and grill the patties for 4 minutes per side until cooked through.

Meanwhile, mix all the feta cheese dressing ingredients in a separate bowl.

Spread the lettuce leaves on four serving plates and top with grilled patties.

Drizzle the feta cheese dressing over them. Garnish with tomato and onion, then serve.

STORAGE: Store in a sealed airtight container in the fridge for up to 2 days or in your freezer for about 1 month.

REHEAT: Microwave, covered, until the desired temperature is reached or reheat in a frying pan or air fryer / instant pot, covered, on medium.

SERVE IT WITH: To add more flavors to this meal, serve this dish with cream cheese dip.

PER SERVING

calories: 320 | fat: 21.0g | total carbs: 6.6g | fiber: 1.3g | protein: 27.6g

Pork Chops with Caramelized Onion

Macros: Fat 60% | Protein 39% | Carbs 1%

Prep time: 10 minutes | Cook time: 30 minutes | Serves 4

With the crispy and crunchy caramelized onion on the side, these pork chops offer a rich mix of flavors. Crispy bacon with creamy sauce makes a balanced combination of flavor, which nicely complements these pork chops.

- 4 ounces (113 g) bacon, chopped
- 1 yellow onion, thinly sliced
- ¼ teaspoon salt
- ¼ teaspoon pepper 4 pork chops
- ½ cup chicken broth
- ¼ cup heavy whipping cream

Heat a large skillet over medium heat until hot.

Add bacon to the hot skillet and cook for 3 to 4 minutes on each side until crispy, then transfer to a bowl. Leave the bacon grease in the skillet.

Toss in onion, along with salt and black pepper, then sauté for 2 minutes until golden brown.

Transfer the sautéed onion to the bacon bowl and keep it aside.

Increase the heat to medium-high and add pork chops.

Sprinkle the salt and black pepper to season the chops. Cook for 5 minutes then flips them. Cook for 6 minutes more until the internal temperature reaches 145°F (63°C).

Remove the chops from the pan and place them on a plate. Cover them

with aluminum sheet and keep them aside.

Pour broth into the same skillet and scrape off the brown bits. Stir in cream and cook for 3 minutes until mixture is thickened.

Return the bacon and onions to the skillet and mix well.

Pour this mixture over the cooked pork chops and serve warm.

STORAGE: Store in a sealed airtight container in the fridge for up to 2 days or in your freezer for about 1 month.

REHEAT: Microwave, covered, until the desired temperature is reached or reheat in a frying pan or instant pot, covered, on medium.

SERVE IT WITH: To add more flavors to this meal, serve the pork chops with cucumber dill cream salad. They also taste great paired with roasted cauliflower florets.

PER SERVING

calories: 485 | fat: 32.4g | total carbs: 1.5g | fiber: 0.2g | protein: 44.2g

Kale Pork Platter with Fried Eggs

Macros: Fat 85% | Protein 10% | Carbs 5%

Prep time: 5 minutes | Cook time: 15 minutes | Serves 4

Now you can enjoy a delicious pork meal in the morning as a breakfast or serve it on the side and make your menu more nutritious and healthier. It has every nutrient that you need on your ketogenic diet. Smoked pork belly with kale and pecans is a combination that you will never forget.

- 3 ounces (85 g) butter
- ½ pound (227 g) kale
- 6 ounces (170 g) smoked pork belly or bacon
- 1 ounce (28 g) pecans or walnuts
- 1 ounce (28 g) frozen cranberries
- 4 eggs
- Salt and black pepper, to taste

Add ⅔ of the butter to a frying pan and melt it over medium-high heat.

Toss in kale leaves and sauté until their edges are slightly browned.

Remove the kale from the pan and keep it in a bowl. Set aside for a while.

Add pork belly to the pan and cook until it is crispy.

Reduce the heat and return the kale to the pan. Add nuts and cranberries and cook for 2 minutes.

Transfer the pork mixture to two serving plates.

Increase the heat and melt the remaining butter in the frying pan.

Crack the eggs one at a time into the pan and fry for about 3 minutes until set.

Top each plate of the pork and kale mixture with two fried eggs. Season as desired with salt and pepper. Serve while still warm.

STORAGE: Store in a sealed airtight container in the fridge for 1 day.

SERVE IT WITH: To add more flavors to this meal, serve this dish with the sliced avocados on top.

PER SERVING

calories: 533 | fat: 49.1g | total carbs: 7.8g | fiber: 2.8g | protein: 17.2g

FISH

Classic Shrimp Scampi

Macros: Fat 9% | Protein 88% | Carbs 3%

Prep time:30 minutes | Cook time: 15 minutes | Serves 4

A restaurant-quality seafood dish that will impress even the pickiest of eaters! These shrimps are sautéed in garlic, butter, and dry white wine, and best enjoyed immediately.

- 2 cloves garlic, minced
- ½ cup butter, melted
- ½ cup dry white wine
- 2 pounds (907 g) medium shrimp, peeled and deveined
- 3 green onions, chopped

Preheat the oven to 400°F (205°C).

In a bowl, combine the garlic, butter, wine, and shrimp. Stir thoroughly.

Arrange the shrimp in a greased baking dish. Place the baking dish in the oven and bake for about 8 minutes until the shrimp is opaque.

Remove from the oven and serve the shrimp with green onions on top.

STORAGE: Store in an airtight container in the fridge for up to 3 to 4 days or in the freezer for up to 1 month.

REHEAT: Microwave, covered, until the desired temperature is reached or reheat in a frying pan or air fryer / instant pot, covered, on medium.

SERVE IT WITH: To make this a complete meal, serve with cauliflower rice.

PER SERVING

calories: 209 | fat: 2.2g | total carbs: 1.6g | fiber: 0.2g | protein: 45.9g

Snow Crab Clusters with Garlic Butter

Macros: Fat 16% | Protein 82% | Carbs 2%

Prep time: 5 minutes | Cook time: 15 minutes | Serves 2

These perfect Crab Clusters with Garlic Butter will melt in your mouth with every bite! The combination of seasonings and succulent taste of the crab will be the only way you'll ever cook crab clusters again!

- 1 pound (454 g) snow crab clusters, thawed if necessary
- ¼ cup butter
- clove garlic, minced
- 1½ teaspoons dried parsley
- ⅛ teaspoon salt
- ¼ teaspoon ground black pepper

On the cutting board, cut a slit lengthwise into the shell of each crab. Set aside.

In a skillet, melt the butter over medium heat. Add the garlic and cook for 2 minutes until tender. Add the parsley, salt, and pepper, then cook for 1 minute more. Stir in the crab and simmer for 5 to 6 minutes.

Remove from the heat and serve on a plate.

STORAGE: Store in an airtight container in the fridge for up to 2 days. Not recommend freezing.

REHEAT: Microwave, covered, until it reaches the desired temperature.

SERVE IT WITH: To make this a complete meal, you can serve it with cabbage and asparagus salad.

PER SERVING

calories: 222 | fat: 4.0g | total carbs: 0.8g | fiber: 0.1g | protein: 45.7g

Creamy Salmon Sauce Zoodles

Macros: Fat 66% | Protein 26% | Carbs 8%

Prep time: 15 minutes | Cook time: 15 minutes | Serves 4

It's an enjoyable time to challenge your friends to try this rich recipes. Creamy salmon sauce zoodles will be your challenging game to make, it's easy to make it at all. The winner will take a priceless prize from his friends.

- 2pounds (907 g) zucchini
- Salt and freshly ground black pepper, to taste
- 4 ounces (113 g) cream cheese
- 1 cup heavy whipping cream
- ¼ cup chopped fresh basil
- 1 pound (454 g) smoked salmon
- 1 lime, juiced
- 2 tablespoons olive oil

Cut the zucchini after washing it thoroughly into thin slices with a sharp knife.

Prepare a colander to filter the zucchini, add a little salt and toss to coat well. Leave them sit for 7 to 12 minutes. Gently press the mixture to get rid of excess salted water.

Meanwhile, mix the cream cheese with lemon juice, chopped fresh basil in a bowl. Set aside until ready to serve.

Cut the salmon into thin slices and sprinkle with salt and pepper. Add the salmon to an oiled skillet and fry over medium-high heat for 8 minutes or until the salmon is opaque and tender on both sides. Then add zucchini spirals and cook for 2 minutes until soft.

Serve the recipe on a large plate with the cream sauce.

STORAGE: We can store extras or the leftovers of this recipe in an airtight container in the refrigerator for up to 5 days, because the recipe contains fish and it will go off if it exceeds this period.

REHEAT: To keep the salmon moist, reheat it inside a foil with a little of olive oil for 5 to 8 minutes in the oven.

SERVE IT WITH: Serve it warm with Italian Sausage and Zucchini Soup or with Creamy Paprika Pork.

PER SERVING

calories: 444 | fat: 33.4g | total carbs: 10.1g | fiber: 2.6g | protein: 29.3g

Delicious Keto Ceviche

Macros: Fat 39% | Protein 50% | Carbs 11%

Prep time: 15 minutes | Cook time: 0 minutes | Serves 4

What a colorful fish! You always have plenty of time to make this easy but incredible recipe. ceviche with its simple ingredient will make your table full of splendid colors.

- 1 pound (454 g) skinless white fish, cut into ½-inch cubes
- ½ red onion, thinly sliced
- 1 fresh jalapeño, deseeded and thinly sliced
- ¼ red bell pepper, thinly sliced
- 1 tablespoon salt
- ¾ cup lime juice, plus more as needed

FOR SERVING:

- 2 tablespoons lime juice
- 1 lime, cut into wedges
- 2 tablespoons olive oil
- 4 tablespoons fresh cilantro, minced

Prepare a dish with a lid to put the skinless white fish, then add the onions, jalapeño, thinly sliced bell pepper, and salt. Toss to coat the fish well. Pour the lime juice over.

Leave the fish in the fridge for about 3 hours for infusing.

Take the fish and vegetables out of the fridge and discard the marinade.

Rinse the fish and vegetables thoroughly with cold water.

Place the fish on a serving dish, then drizzle with olive oil and lemon juice. Spread the fresh cilantro for topping. Serve cold with lime.

STORAGE: You can easily store extras or the leftovers of keto ceviche in an airtight bag in the freezer for up to 3 days.

SERVE IT WITH: Serve it chilled with creamy paprika pork to let your dinner perfect.

PER SERVING

calories: 174 | fat:7.6g | total carbs: 6.3g | fiber: 0.6g | protein: 20.7g

Cabbage Plate with Keto Salmon

Macros: Fat 73% | Protein 12% | Carbs 16%

Prep time: 5 minutes | Cook time: 0 minutes | Serves 4

You do not have enough time to prepare dinner after work, confused about the recipe you want to prepare. Don't worry! With the avocado plate with cream salmon, you can amaze you with its great taste. With only four ingredients, you can prepare a cool, speedy, and splendid dinner!

- 7 ounces (198 g) fresh salmon
- 2 avocados
- 2 teaspoons coconut oil
- 6 teaspoons olive oil, divided
- ½ teaspoon onion powder,
- 1 teaspoon turmeric
- 2 cups shredded coconut, unsweetened
- 12 ounces (340 g) cabbage, chopped
- 2 teaspoons butter
- 1 pinch of lemon zest
- Salt and freshly ground black pepper, to taste

Cut the salmon into 1×1-inch pieces. Then drizzle the coconut oil and 2 teaspoons of olive oil on salmon pieces. Place the pieces in a medium bowl and set aside.

Mix the salt, onion powder, turmeric, and unsweetened shredded coconut in a separate bowl. Meanwhile, dunk the pre-prepared salmon pieces into this mixture.

In a nonstick frying pan with 4 teaspoons of olive oil on medium heat. Fry the seasoned salmon pieces with coconut mixture for about 4 to 7 minutes in a pan, stirring every 2 minutes. Leave it in the pan until golden brown and soft.

Meanwhile, fry the cabbage in a saucepan with butter until it is lightly caramelized. In a third bowl, pour the cabbage liquid and generously season with salt and pepper.

On a dish with lemon slices, place the fried salmon and pour the creamy cabbage over it. Serve warm.

STORAGE: Store in an airtight container in the fridge for up to 4 days or in the freezer for up to 1 month.

REHEAT: You can reheat the extras in a light skillet on medium-low heat until warmed through.

SERVE IT WITH: Serve it immediately with roasted vegetable soup or avocado crunchy fries to be a splendid meal.

PER SERVING

calories: 502 | fat: 42.8g | total carbs: 21.2g | fiber: 12.7g | protein: 14.8g

Asparagus Seared Salmon with Easy Hollandaise

Macros: Fat 74% | Protein 23% | Carbs 3%

Prep time: 10 minutes | Cook time: 20 minutes | Serves 4

Do you watch movies with your friends, but feel very boring! Try eating asparagus Seared salmon with easy Hollandaise while watching your favorite movies and you will feel the difference. It can be prepared fast and easily with your friends at your sweet home.

- 1 tablespoon butter
- 20 ounces (567 g) salmon fillets
- Salt and freshly ground black pepper, to taste
- 14 ounces (397 g) green asparagus, rinsed and trimmed

HOLLANDAISE:

- 1 egg
- 7 ounces (198 g) butter, melted
- 1 tablespoon lemon juice
- 1 lemon, sliced

Melt the butter in a large skillet over medium heat.

Add the salmon fillets and cook for 14 minutes or until opaque. Flip the fillets halfway through the cooking time.

Add the asparagus gradually to the skillet while cooking the fillets and season with salt and pepper. Sauté the asparagus for 10 minutes or until soft and wilted.

Reduce the heat to low to keep the salmon and asparagus warm while making the Hollandaise..

HOLLANDAISE:

Break the egg in a bowl, then melt the butter in the microwave

Pour slowly melted butter into the egg in the mixing bowl. Keep stirring to mix until creamy.

Add lemon juice and salt.

Serve the salmon with creamy Hollandaise and soft asparagus. Decorate with slices of lemon for extra flavor and color.

STORAGE: Store the leftovers of salmon in an airtight container in the fridge for up to 5 days or in the freezer for up to 1 month.

REHEAT: You can reheat the extras in a lightly oiled skillet on medium-low heat until the salmon moistened through.

SERVE IT WITH: To make this a complete meal, you can serve it with roasted cauliflower.

PER SERVING

calories: 639 | fat: 53.7g | total carbs: 5.3g | fiber: 2.2g | protein: 35.2g

SOUPS

Garlicky Pork Soup with Cauliflower and Tomatoes

Macros: Fat: 45% | Protein: 48% | Carbs: 7%

Prep time: 20 minutes | Cook time: 45 minutes | Serves 8

This garlicky pork soup dish is a comforting, hearty, flavorful dish for everyone. Made under an hour, it is a quick and easy no-fuss soup perfect for everyday cooking.

- 2 pounds (907 g) boneless pork ribs, cut into 1-inch pieces
- 2 tablespoons olive oil
- 1 tablespoon garlic, chopped
- ½ cup onions, chopped
- ½ cup dry white wine
- 1 cup chicken stock
- 1 cup of water
- 2 cups fresh tomatoes, chopped
- 2 cups cauliflower, finely chopped
- 2 tablespoons fresh oregano, chopped
- Salt and freshly ground black pepper, to taste

Generously sprinkle the pork with salt and pepper.

Heat the olive oil in a pan over medium heat and add the pork. Cook for 3 minutes on each side until it is brown, then add the garlic and the onions.

Cook for 2 minutes then add the wine, chicken stock, water, and tomatoes.

Let it boil, then pour it into a crockpot to cook on high for 4 hours.

Mix in the cauliflower and the oregano, then let it cook for 20 minutes more.

Serve immediately.

STORAGE: Store in an airtight container in the fridge for up to 4 days or in the freezer for up to 1 month.

REHEAT: Microwave, covered, until the desired temperature is reached or reheat in a frying pan or instant pot, covered, on medium.

SERVE IT WITH: To make this a complete meal, serve it with Parmesan roasted zucchini.

PER SERVING

calories: 210 | fat: 10.4g | total carbs: 6.5g | fiber: 1.8g | protein: 25.5g

Cheesy Zucchini Soup

Macros: Fat: 82% | Protein: 10% | Carbs: 8%

Prep time: 2 hours | Cook time: 10 minutes | Serves 5

This quick and easy soup is perfect for busy weekdays and nights. With ingredients you already have in your kitchen, each bite of this delicious low- carb soup helps you feel relaxed and comfortable in your home.

- 4 cups chicken broth
- 1 medium zucchini, cut into ½-inch pieces
- 8 ounces (227 g) cream cheese cut into cubes
- ½ teaspoon ground cumin
- Salt and black pepper, to taste

SPECIAL EQUIPMENT:

Immersion blender

Pour the chicken broth into a large pot and add the zucchini. Boil for 5 minutes then reduce the heat and simmer for 10 minutes.

Mix in the cream cheese, then remove the pot from the heat. Blend the soup with an immersion blender until it is smooth, then add the cumin, salt, and pepper.

Put it in the refrigerator for 2 hours to chill.

Serve the soup into bowls.

STORAGE: Store in an airtight container in the fridge for up to 4 days or in the freezer for up to 1 month.

REHEAT: Microwave, covered, until the desired temperature is reached or reheat in a frying pan or instant pot, covered, on medium.

PER SERVING

calories: 178 | fat: 16.1g | total carbs: 4.1g | fiber: 0.4g | protein: 4.5g

Creamy Veggie Soup

Prep time: 20 minutes | Cook time: 10 minutes | Serves 7
Macros: Fat: 69% | Protein: 11% | Carbs: 20%

This creamy veggie dish is the perfect low-carb soup for everyone. Made with a variety of healthy ingredients and spices, this dish is quick and easy to make and will give you enough energy to stay on top of your daily activities.

- ¼ cup butter
- 1 medium white onion, diced
- 2 garlic cloves
- 1 medium head cauliflower
- 1 bay leaf, crumbled
- 7 ounces (198 g) fresh spinach
- 5 ounces (142 g) watercress
- 4 cups vegetable stock
- 1 cup coconut cream
- Salt and freshly ground black pepper, to taste

SPECIAL EQUIPMENT:

Immersion blender

Heat the butter in a pot over medium heat and add the onions and garlic.

Cook until it is golden brown.

Mix in the cauliflower and the bay leaf, then let it cook for 5 minutes.

Add the spinach and the watercress. Cook for another 3 minutes, then pour in the stock and let it boil.

Add the coconut cream and sprinkle it with salt and pepper. Remove the pot from the heat.

Puree with an immersion blender until it is smooth, then put it in the refrigerator to chill for 1 hour.

Serve chilled.

STORAGE: Store in an airtight container in the fridge for up to 4 days or in the freezer for up to 1 month.

REHEAT: Microwave, covered, until the desired temperature is reached or reheat in a frying pan or instant pot, covered, on medium.

SERVE IT WITH: To make this a complete meal, serve it with some warm keto bread.

PER SERVING

calories: 259 | fat: 20.0g | total carbs: 18.0g | fiber: 5.1g | protein: 6.9g

Creamy and Cheesy Spicy Avocado Soup

Macros: Fat: 80% | Protein: 10% | Carbs: 10%

Prep time: 5 minutes | Cook time: 10 minutes | Serves 6

What dish is better than guacamole? This creamy and cheesy guacamole soup is the right answer. This avocado soup dish is the perfect soup dish for all guacamole lovers, made with spicy and creamy ingredients, this soup dish will take you on a gooey ride your taste buds will not want to return from.

- 2 avocados, peeled and pitted
- ¼ cup red onion, chopped
- 1 tablespoon fresh cilantro, chopped
- 2½ cups low-sodium chicken broth, divided
- 2 garlic cloves, coarsely chopped
- 1 jalapeño, seeded and coarsely chopped
- 1 tablespoon lime juice
- ¼ teaspoon black pepper
- ½ teaspoon salt
- ¼ teaspoon cayenne
- ¼ cup whipping cream
- 2 tablespoons sour cream
- 6 tablespoons Cheddar cheese, shredded

Put the avocado, onion, cilantro, 1 cup of the chicken broth, garlic, jalapeño, and lime juice into a food processor and pulse until it is smooth.

Add the rest of the broth, black pepper, salt, cayenne, and whipping cream to the food processor and pulse again until it is creamy, then pour it into a bowl.

Put the bowl in the refrigerator to chill for 1 hour.

Serve the soup into bowls topped with sour cream and Cheddar cheese.

STORAGE: Store in an airtight container in the fridge for up to 4 days or in the freezer for up to 1 month.

REHEAT: Microwave, covered, until the desired temperature is reached or reheat in a frying pan or instant pot, covered, on medium.

SERVE IT WITH: To make this a complete meal, serve it with roasted zucchini sticks.

PER SERVING

calories: 185 | fat: 16.4g | total carbs: 9.4g | fiber: 4.7g | protein: 4.6g

Creamy Minty Spinach Soup

Macros: Fat: 68% | Protein: 15% | Carbs: 17%

Prep time: 5 minutes | Cook time: 10 minutes | Serves 3

This creamy minty spinach soup is filling and healthy. It is delicious and nutritious and perfect for any time of the year. It is quick and easy and is great for lunch or dinner. Kick back and let your taste buds run wild.

- 1 tablespoon olive oil
- 4 spring onions, chopped
- 2 garlic cloves
- 12 ounces (340 g) spinach leaves
- 1½ cups chicken stock
- ½ cup mint leaves
- 4 tablespoons heavy cream
- Salt and black pepper, to taste

Heat the oil in a pot over medium heat and add the onions and garlic.

Cook for 3 minutes then add the spinach leaves.

Let it cook for 4 minutes, then add the stock and mint leaves, then pour it into a blender.

Pulse until it is smooth, then mix in the heavy cream, salt, and pepper.

Put it in the refrigerator to chill until ready to serve.

Serve chilled.

STORAGE: Store in an airtight container in the fridge for up to 4 days or in the freezer for up to 1 month.

REHEAT: Microwave, covered, until the desired temperature is reached or reheat in a frying pan or instant pot, covered, on medium.

SERVE IT WITH: To make this a complete meal, serve it with some warm keto bread.

PER SERVING

calories: 184 | fat: 13.9g | total carbs: 10.8g | fiber: 3.1g | protein: 7.1g

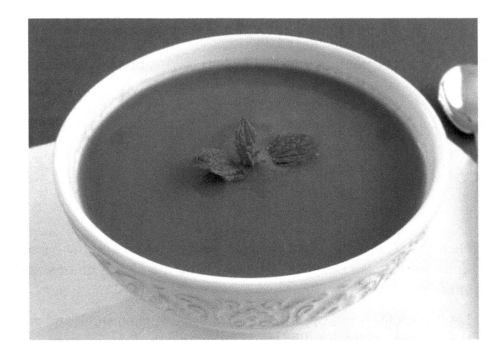

Creamy Chicken and Bacon Chipotle Soup

Macros: Fat: 68% | Protein: 26% | Carbs: 6%

Prep time: 13 minutes | Cook time: 20 minutes | Serves 8

This mouthwatering chicken and bacon chipotle soup is the perfect dish for cold nights. Quick and easy to make. This dish is perfect for lunch or dinner for everyone. It is guaranteed to make every table a loving one.

- 1 tablespoon olive oil
- 6 bacon slices, chopped
- 1 medium onion, chopped
- 2 garlic cloves, minced
- 3 cups chicken stock
- 1¼ pounds (567 g) chicken thighs, boneless, skinless, cut into 1-inch chunks
- 1 teaspoon salt
- ½ teaspoon black pepper
- 2 cups heavy cream
- 1 chipotle pepper in adobo, minced
- 2 tablespoons fresh cilantro, chopped

Heat the olive oil in a pan over medium heat and add the bacon. Cook until it is crispy for 5 minutes, then add the onions and garlic.

Let it cook for 3 minutes, then pour in the chicken stock and add the chicken. Boil for 3 minutes then reduce the temperature.

Cook on low for 10 minutes, then season it with salt and black pepper.

Mix in the heavy cream and chipotle and let it cook for 5 minutes.

Serve into bowls sprinkled with fresh cilantro.

STORAGE: Store in an airtight container in the fridge for up to 4 days or in the freezer for up to 1 month.

REHEAT: Microwave, covered, until the desired temperature is reached or reheat in a frying pan or instant pot, covered, on medium.

PER SERVING

calories: 363 | fat: 27.3g | total carbs: 6.4g | fiber: 0.4g | protein: 23.2g

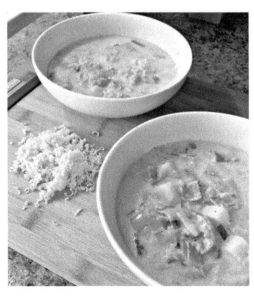

Cheesy Turkey and Bacon Soup with Celery and Parsley

Macros: Fat: 50% | Protein: 41% | Carbs: 9%

Prep time: 7 minutes | Cook time: 33 minutes | Serves 8

This mouthwatering turkey and bacon soup with celery and parsley is the perfect soup combination for all poultry and meat lovers. This delicious soup is quick and easy to make, especially during busy weekdays and nights. It can be eaten whether during lunch or dinner and stores perfectly to be eaten at a later date.

- 1 tablespoon olive oil
- 8 ounces (227 g) bacon, crumbled
- 1 large shallot, peeled and chopped
- ½ cup celery, chopped
- 4 cups cooked turkey meat, shredded or chopped
- 8 cups turkey (or chicken) stock
- ½ cup heavy whipping cream
- ½ cup extra sharp Cheddar cheese, shredded
- 1 teaspoon dried parsley
- ½ teaspoon liquid smoke
- 1 teaspoon xanthan gum
- 1 tablespoon fresh thyme leaves
- Salt and freshly ground black pepper, to taste

Heat the olive oil in a pot over medium heat, then add the bacon, shallots, and celery. Cook for 5 minutes.

Pour in the turkey meat, turkey stock, whipping cream, and add the Cheddar cheese. Cook for 3 minutes.

Mix in the parsley and liquid smoke, then let it cook on low heat for 20 minutes.

Add the xanthan gum and whisk it well, then let it cook for 5 minutes.

Mix in the fresh thyme, then season with salt and black pepper.

Serve into bowls while it is hot.

STORAGE: Store in an airtight container in the fridge for up to 4 days or in the freezer for up to 1 month.

REHEAT: Microwave, covered, until the desired temperature is reached or reheat in a frying pan or instant pot, covered, on medium.

PER SERVING

calories: 461 | fat: 25.7g | total carbs: 10.2g | fiber: 0.2g | protein: 47.5g

Spicy Shrimp and Veggies Cream Soup

Macros: Fat: 64% | Protein: 27% | Carbs: 9%

Prep time: 5 minutes | Cook time: 40 minutes | Serves 8

This creamy shrimp and veggie soup are for seafood lovers who enjoy that spicy flavor on their tongues when they eat their favorite seafood soup. This delicious soup is perfect for all ages and serves easily as a lunch or dinner meal.

- 2 tablespoons avocado oil
- ¼ cup onions, diced
- Salt and freshly ground black pepper, to taste
- 2 celery stalks chopped
- 1 jalapeño, seeded and diced
- 2 tablespoons green Thai curry paste
- 1 (15-ounce / 425-g) can unsweetened coconut milk
- 3 cups chicken broth
- ½ head cabbage, roughly chopped
- ½ pound (227 g) raw shrimp peeled and deveined
- 1 pound (454 g) wild Pacific cod cut into 1-inch chunks
- 2 tablespoons fresh lime juice
- 2 tablespoons fish sauce
- ¼ cup fresh cilantro, chopped

Heat the oil in a pan over medium heat and add the onion, salt, and pepper. Cook for 4 minutes then add the celery and jalapeño.

Cook for 3 minutes then add the curry paste and cook for 30 seconds.

Pour in the coconut milk and the broth.

Add the cabbage and cook on low heat for 10 minutes.

Mix in the shrimp and cod chunks. Cook for 10 minutes again.

Remove from the heat and mix in the lime juice and fish sauce.

Serve the soup into bowls topped with fresh cilantro.

STORAGE: Store in an airtight container in the fridge for up to 4 days or in the freezer for up to 1 month.

REHEAT: Microwave, covered, until the desired temperature is reached or reheat in a frying pan or instant pot, covered, on medium.

SERVE IT WITH: To make this a complete meal, serve it with a bowl of salad.

PER SERVING

calories: 250 | fat: 17.6g | total carbs: 8.0g | fiber: 2.2g | protein: 17.1g

SALADS

Feta Cheese and Cucumber Salad

Macros: Fat 80% | Protein 9% | Carbs 11%

Prep time: 10 minutes | Cook time: 0 minutes | Serves 5

Share this amazing feta cheese and cucumber salad with your family, especially on a sunny afternoon. To enjoy the salad, chill before serving, although you can take the salad immediately after preparation.

SALAD:

- 2medium cucumbers
- ½ cup thinly sliced red onions
- 4 ounces (113 g) feta cheese, crumbled
- Salt and freshly ground black pepper, to taste

DRESSING:

- ¼ cup extra-virgin olive oil
- 1 tablespoon Swerve
- 1 tablespoon red wine vinegar
- ½ teaspoon dried ground oregano

Peel the cucumbers to your preference. On your cutting board, cut them in half lengthwise and then slice.

Put the sliced cucumbers in a large bowl, then add the onions and toss fully. Sprinkle with the feta cheese and combine well. Set aside.

Meanwhile, start the dressing by putting all the ingredients for dressing in another bowl, then whisk thoroughly to incorporate.

Pour the dressing into the bowl of cucumber salad and toss well. Season as desired with salt and pepper before serving.

STORAGE: Store in a separate airtight container in the fridge for up to 3 days.

SERVE IT WITH: To make this a complete meal, you can serve it with grilled chicken or fish fillets.

PER SERVING

calories: 177 | fat: 15.8g | total carbs: 5.7g | fiber: 0.8g | protein: 3.8g

Ranch Chicken and Bacon Salad

Macros: Fat 86% | Protein 13% | Carbs 1%

Prep time: 10 minutes | Cook time: 10 minutes | Serves 6

A salad made up of chicken can be taken for lunch or dinner. The combination of bacon, chicken, and vegetables equals to a tasty and nutritious meal. You can choose to garnish the salad with freshly chopped parsley or serve without the parsley.

- 5 slices bacon
- 12 ounces (340 g) cubed cooked chicken
- ½ chopped stalk celery
- ⅓ cup keto-friendly mayonnaise
- 3 tablespoons ranch dressing
- Salt and freshly ground pepper, to taste
- 6 butterhead lettuce leaves, for serving

Fry the bacon in a skillet over medium heat for 8 minutes until crispy, then transfer to a plate lined with paper towels. When cool enough to handle, crumble the bacon into smaller pieces with a spatula.

In a medium bowl, put the cooked chicken. Add the celery, mayonnaise, ranch dressing, and bacon pieces. Using a fork to stir the mixture until well combined. Sprinkle the salt and pepper to season.

Evenly divide the salad on the lettuce leaves and serve immediately.

STORAGE: Store in separate airtight containers in the fridge for up to 3 days.

SERVE IT WITH: To make this a complete meal, you can serve it with broccoli soup.

PER SERVING

calories: 469 | fat: 45.2g | total carbs: 0.8g | fiber: 0.1g | protein: 14.4g

Grilled Salmon and Greek Salad

Macros: Fat 55% | Protein 32% | Carbs 13%

Prep time: 15 minutes | Cook time: 10 minutes | Serves 4

Grilled salmon when served with a chilled salad is so satisfying. The salad is perfect for the evenings where you get home tired and just want something easy to fix. Within a few minutes, you will have your complete meal.

SALAD:

- 2 medium heads Romaine lettuce, chopped
- ½ medium cucumber, chopped
- ¾ cup feta cheese, crumbled
- ¾ cup cherry tomatoes, halved
- ½ cup red onions, thinly sliced
- ½ cup Kalamata olives, pitted
- 1 teaspoon dried ground oregano
- Salt and freshly ground black pepper, to taste

DRESSING:

- 2 teaspoons dried ground oregano
- 2 tablespoons extra-virgin olive oil
- 2 teaspoons onion powder
- 1 large clove garlic, minced
- ¼ cup red wine vinegar
- Salt and freshly ground black pepper, to taste

SALMON:

- 4 (6-ounce / 170-g) skin-on salmon fillets, rinsed and drained
- 1 tablespoon extra-virgin olive oil
- Salt and freshly ground black pepper, to taste
- 1 tablespoon avocado oil, for greasing the grill grates
  Fresh dill, for garnish

Put all the ingredients for salad in a large bowl and toss to combine well.

Divide the salad into four serving bowls and put aside.

In the meantime, make the dressing by adding the oregano, olive oil, onion powder, garlic, pepper, salt, and vinegar in another bowl. Stir thoroughly, then put aside.

Brush the salmon with olive oil on both sides, then season with pepper and salt to taste.

Preheat the grill to medium-high heat, then grease the grill grates with avocado oil.

Grill the salmon for 3 minutes, skin facing up. Turn the salmon over and grill for about 5 minutes, or until the internal temperature reads 145 □ (63 □).

Let the salmon rest for about 5 minutes, then put the fillets on top of the salad in four serving bowls. Pour the dressing over the salads and sprinkle the fresh dill on top for garnish before serving.

STORAGE: Store in separate airtight containers in the fridge for up to 3 days.

REHEAT: Microwave the salmon, covered, until the desired temperature is reached.

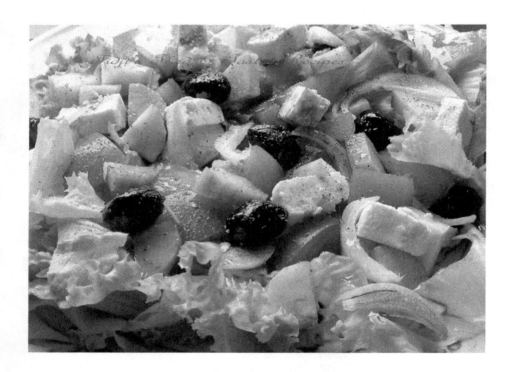

Simple Cauliflower Salad

Macros: Fat 75% | Protein 11% | Carbs 15%

Prep time: 15 minutes | Cook time: 5 minutes | Serves 2

Enjoy the tasty cauliflower salad made with a variety of other vegetables. The grated Parmesan cheese gives the meal a unique taste that will leave you wanting more. If you love bacon, you can enjoy the salad with some bacon strips.

- ½ cup chopped cauliflower
- ⅛ cup chopped fresh basil
- ¾ tablespoon chopped kalamata olives
- ½ minced garlic clove
- ¾ tablespoon chopped sun-dried tomatoes
- ⅛ cup grated Cheddar cheese
- ¾ tablespoon balsamic vinegar
- ¾ tablespoon extra-virgin olive oil
- Salt and freshly ground black pepper, to taste

Microwave the chopped cauliflower for 5 minutes or until just tender.

Meanwhile, in a mixing bowl, combine the basil, olives, garlic, tomatoes, and cheese. Add the cooked cauliflower and toss well.

In another bowl, whisk together the vinegar and olive oil. Pour the mixture over the cauliflower mixture. Sprinkle with salt and pepper and stir well before serving.

STORAGE: Store in separate airtight containers in the fridge for up to 3 days.

SERVE IT WITH: To make this a complete meal, serve the cauliflower salad with crispy bacon slices.

PER SERVING

calories: 101 | fat: 8.4g | total carbs: 4.0g | fiber: 1.0g | protein: 3.0g

Kale and Avocado Salad with Lemon Dijon Vinaigrette Dressing

Macros: Fat 85% | Protein 3% | Carbs 11%

Prep time: 25 minutes | Cook time: 15 minutes | Serves 4

The Kale and Avocado Salad is the perfect match for keto diet, especially when it is flavored with the Lemon Dijon Vinaigrette dressing. I personally tried it and it tastes amazingly good.

DRESSING:

- 1½ tablespoons Dijon mustard
- 2 tablespoons lemon juice
- ¼ teaspoon ground black pepper
- Sea salt, to taste
- ¼ cup olive oil

SALAD:

- 1 bundle kale, torn into small pieces
- ½ avocado, sliced
- ½ cup cucumber, chopped
- ⅔ cup cherry tomatoes, quartered
- 2 tablespoons red onion, chopped finely
- ⅓ cup red bell pepper, chopped finely
- 1 tablespoon feta cheese

In a bowl, mix Dijon mustard, lemon juice, black pepper, sea salt and olive oil together until well combined. Set aside.

Blanch the kale in a saucepan of salted water for about 45 seconds until hot.

Remove from the heat to a plate. Put the avocado, cucumber, cherry tomatoes, onion, bell pepper and feta cheese on top.

Pour the mustard mixture over the salad and toss well, then serve.

STORAGE: The salad can be stored covered in the fridge for 3 to 5 days.

SERVE IT WITH: The Kale and Avocado Salad can be a side dish with any other main dishes.

PER SERVING

calories: 187 | fat: 18.3g | total carbs: 5.8g | fiber: 2.8g | protein: 1.9g

Low-Carb Dressing

Macros: Fat 98% | Protein 1% | Carbs 1%

Prep time: 10 minutes | Cook time: 0 minutes | Serves 6

Looking for a dip or dressing that is keto-friendly? This low-carb dressing perfectly pairs with your keto-friendly salads.

* ¼ cup keto-friendly mayonnaise
* ¼ cup olive oil
* 2 tablespoons MTC oil
* 1 tablespoon Dijon mustard
* 2 cloves garlic, peeled and crushed
* 2 tablespoons lemon juice
* 2 tablespoons fresh parsley, chopped finely
* Himalayan pink salt and ground black pepper, to taste

In a jar, mix together mayonnaise, olive oil, MCT oil, Dijon mustard, garlic and lemon juice.

Add chopped parsley, salt and pepper. Tightly cover the jar, then shake until well combined, then serve.

STORAGE: This keto dressing can be stored in an airtight container in the refrigerator for about 1 week. You can store it in the freezer for up to 1 month.

SERVE IT WITH: The keto dressing can be served as a dip, or mix with salad greens.

PER SERVING

calories: 198 | fat: 21.5g | total carbs: 1.0g | fiber: 0.2g | protein: 0.3g

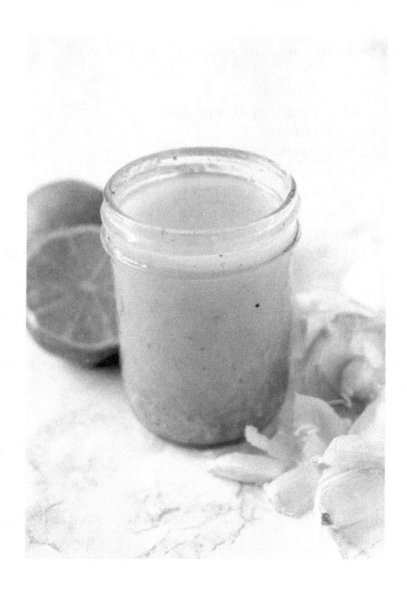

Keto Quick Caesar Dressing

Macros: Fat 87% | Protein 8% | Carbs 5%

Prep time: 5 minutes | Cook time: 0 minutes | Serves 4

To enjoy your meal to the utmost, try to prepare this keto quick Caesar dressing. Cool yourself down with this cheesy buttered to put it in your dinner, lunch or even supper.

- 1½ ounces (42 g) Parmesan cheese, grated
- ¼ cup olive oil
- 1 tablespoon Dijon mustard
- 1 teaspoon red wine vinegar
- 1 pinch ground black pepper
- ½ garlic clove, minced
- ½ teaspoon salt
- ½ lemon, the juice

Whisk the Parmesan cheese, olive oil, mustard, wine vinegar, pepper, garlic well in a bowl except for the salt, until smooth, add salt and pepper to taste. Keep stirring.

To reduce the density of the mixture, gradually add about a teaspoon of water or lemon juice at a time to obtain the desired consistency.

STORAGE: Store the left dressing in an airtight container in the fridge for 5 days, and it can also be kept in the freezer for 30 days. It can serve with any meal.

SERVE IT WITH: Serve it with crunchy vegetables, high-fat cheese or serve it with a dish of warm Broccoli Cheddar Soup.

PER SERVING

calories: 169 | fat: 16.6g | total carbs: 2.3g | fiber: 0.2g | protein: 3.2g

Mediterranean Baked Spinach with Cheese

Macros: Fat 75% | Protein 13% | Carbs 11%

Prep time: 5 minutes | Cook time: 25 minutes | Serves 6

Spinach gets a Mediterranean touch when baked in a casserole with a mixture of feta cheese with pitted black olives and butter. The recipe is easy to follow and takes a short time to prepare.

- 2 tablespoons olive oil
- 2 cups water
- 2 pounds (907 g) chopped spinach
- 4 tablespoons butter
- Salt and black pepper, to taste
- 1½ cups grated feta cheese
- ½ cup halved and pitted black olives
- 4 teaspoons grated fresh lemon zest

Preheat the air fryer to 400°F (205°C) and grease the air fryer basket with olive oil.

In a pan, add water and bring to a boil. Add the spinach and blanch for about 4 minutes. Drain the excess water.

In a bowl, add the spinach, butter, salt, and black pepper and mix. Transfer to the air fryer basket and cook for 15 minutes. Stir once halfway through the cooking time.

Transfer to serving bowls and add the cheese, olives, and lemon zest. Stir well before serving.

STORAGE: Store in an airtight container in the fridge for up to 3 days.

SERVE IT WITH: If you are a meat lover, you can enjoy this dish with roast chicken breasts or garlicky shrimp skewers; if you are a vegan, then you can serve it with a cup of green smoothie or a green salad.

PER SERVING

calories: 254 | fat: 21.9g | total carbs: 7.9g | fiber: 3.7g | protein: 9.8g

Cheesy Cauliflower Bake

Macros: Fat 82% | Protein 9% | Carbs 9%

Prep time: 5 minutes | Cook time: 30 minutes | Serves 6

The cheesy cauliflower recipe takes a quick time to prepare. The cheesy cauliflower is a delicious way to make a low-carb and keto-friendly side dish that's packed with vegetables.

- 2 tablespoons olive oil
- 2 teaspoons avocado mayonnaise, keto-friendly
- 2 tablespoons mustard
- 2 chopped cauliflower heads
- ½ cup butter, chopped into ½-inch pieces
- 1 cup grated Parmesan cheese

Preheat the oven to 400°F (205°C) and grease a baking dish with olive oil.

In a bowl, add the avocado mayonnaise and mustard and mix well. Coat cauliflower heads with this mixture before placing in the baking dish.

Top with butter and Parmesan cheese and bake in the preheated oven until the cauliflower heads are soft for 25 minutes.

Transfer to serving plates to cool before serving.

STORAGE: Store in an airtight container in the fridge for up to 4 days or in the freezer for up to 1 month.

REHEAT: Microwave, covered, until it reaches the desired temperature.

SERVE IT WITH: To make this a complete meal, serve with Turmeric Beef Bone Broth.

PER SERVING

calories: 282 | fat: 26.2g | total carbs: 7.0g | fiber: 2.0g | protein: 6.8g

Easy Parmesan Roasted Bamboo Sprouts

Macros: Fat 67% | Protein 17% | Carbs 16%

Prep time: 8 minutes | Cook time: 15 minutes | Serves6

Parmesan roasted bamboo sprouts are vegetarian-friendly and gluten-free. Pepper is added to the treat to spice it up. It takes a short time to prepare.

- 2 tablespoons olive oil
- 2 pounds (907 g) bamboo shoots
- ½ teaspoon paprika
- Salt and black pepper, to taste
- 4 tablespoons butter
- 2 cups grated Parmesan cheese

Preheat the oven to 375°F (190°C) and grease a baking dish with olive oil.

Combine the bamboo shoots with paprika, salt, black pepper, and butter in a large bowl. Wrap the bowl in plastic and refrigerate to marinate for at least 1 hour.

Discard the marinade and transfer the bamboo sprouts to the baking dish and bake in the preheated oven for 15 minutes.

Transfer to serving plates to cool and top with cheese before serving.

STORAGE: Store in an airtight container in the fridge for up to 4 days or in the freezer for up to 1 month.

REHEAT: Microwave, covered, until it reaches the desired temperature.

SERVE IT WITH: To make this a complete meal, serve with chicken stuffed avocados.

PER SERVING

calories: 289 | fat: 21.9g | total carbs: 12.6g | fiber: 3.4g | protein: 13.5g

Cauliflower Bread Sticks with Cheese

Macros: Fat 76% | Protein 21% | Carbs 3%

Prep time: 10 minutes | Cook time: 20minutes | Serves 2

The delicacy is gluten-free, low-carb and very simple to make. The treat has a very direct recipe that takes a short time to prepare. The crust can also be used for making pizza.

- 1 tablespoon olive oil
- ½ cup riced cauliflower
- ⅛ teaspoon ground oregano
- ⅛ teaspoon ground sage
- ⅛ teaspoon ground mustard
- ⅛ teaspoon thyme, dried
- 1 small beaten egg
- ½ cup freshly grated Monterey jack cheese
- Salt and ground black pepper, to taste
- Minced fresh parsley, for garnish

In a toaster oven, add the cauliflower and cook for 8 minutes or until soft.

In a bowl, add the cooked cauliflower. Add the oregano, sage, mustard, and thyme for seasoning.

Add the egg, ½ of cheese, salt and black pepper.

Preheat the oven to 450°F (235°C) and grease a baking sheet with olive oil.

Arrange the cauliflower mixture on the greased baking sheet.

Bake in the preheated oven for 8 minutes. Top with remaining cheese and bake for an additional 5 minutes or until the cheese melts.

Remove from oven, garnish with parsley, and slice into sticks before serving

STORAGE: Store in an airtight container in the fridge for up to 4 days or in the freezer for up to 1 month.

REHEAT: Microwave, covered, until it reaches the desired temperature.

SERVE IT WITH: To make this a complete meal, serve with blackberry chocolate shake.

PER SERVING

calories: 218 | fat: 18.7g | total carbs: 1.8g | fiber: 0.6g | protein: 11.0g

Almond Fritters with Mayo Sauce

Macros: Fat 67% | Protein 18% | Carbs 15%

Prep time: 5 minutes | Cook time: 15 minutes | Serves 2

I know you do fancy fritters. You will realize that the ingredients reveal how nutritious the dish is. You will enjoy the flavors and the cheesy nature of the recipe. You will take less than 20 minutes to prepare the recipe.

FRITTERS:

- 1 ounce (28 g) fresh broccoli
- 1 small whisked egg
- 1 ounce (28 g) Mozzarella cheese
- 2 tablespoons plus
- 1 tablespoon flaxseed meal, divided
- 4 tablespoons almond flour
- ¼ teaspoon baking powder
- Salt and freshly ground black pepper, to taste

SAUCE:

- 4 tablespoons fresh dill, chopped
- 4 tablespoons mayonnaise, keto-friendly
- ½ teaspoon lemon juice
- Salt and freshly ground black pepper, to taste

Make the fritters: In a food processor, add the broccoli and process until chopped thoroughly.

In a bowl, add the processed broccoli, whisked egg, Mozzarella cheese, 2 tablespoons of flaxseed meal, almond flour, baking powder, black pepper and salt. Mix well to form batter. Divide and roll into 4 equal balls.

In a bowl, add the remaining 1 tablespoon of flaxseed meal. Dip the balls in this bowl to coat well.

Preheat an air fryer to 375°F (190°C) and place balls in the basket.

Fry fritters until golden brown for 5 minutes. Transfer to a serving plate.

Make the sauce: In a bowl, add the dill, mayonnaise, lemon juice, salt, and pepper and mix well.

Dip the fritters into the sauce and serve.

STORAGE: Store in an airtight container in the fridge for up to 4 days or in the freezer for up to 1 month.

REHEAT: Microwave, covered, until it reaches the desired temperature.

SERVE IT WITH: To make this a complete meal, serve with keto tropical smoothie.

PER SERVING

calories: 381 | fat: 29.5g | total carbs: 17.7g | fiber: 9.6g | protein: 18.2g

Almond Sausage Balls

Macros: Fat 74% | Proteins 19% | Carbs 7%

Prep time: 30 minutes | Cook time: 25 minutes | Serves 6

With only five ingredients, get into the kitchen and prepare almond sausage balls within a few minutes. Take the keto balls anytime you feel hungry. Prepare in advance to save time. If you have kids, do not miss out on these tasty balls.

* 1 cup almond flour, blanched
* 3 ounces bulk Italian sausage
* 1¼ cups sharp Cheddar cheese, shredded
* 2 teaspoons baking powder
* 1 large egg

Start by preheating the oven to 350°F (180°C) then grease a baking tray.

In a mixing bowl, mix the almond flour, Italian sausage, Cheddar cheese, baking powder, and the egg until mixed evenly.

Make equal-sized balls out of the mixture, then put them on the baking tray.

Put in the oven and bake for 20 minutes or until golden brown.

Remove from the oven and serve.

STORAGE: Store in an airtight container in the fridge for up to 1 week.

REHEAT: Microwave, covered, until it reaches the desired temperature.

PER SERVING

calories: 266 | fat: 22.5g | total carbs: 4.7g | fiber: 2.0g | protein: 13.0g

Cheesy Keto Cupcakes

Macros: Fat 85% | Proteins 9% | Carbs 6%

Prep time: 10 minutes | Cook: 20 minutes | Serves 12

It requires few ingredients when preparing this recipe. Only six ingredients and you have your cupcakes ready. They are soft, tasty and delicious. Good, especially for kids.

- ¼ cup melted butter
- ½ cup almond meal
- 1 teaspoon vanilla extract
- 2 (8-ounce / 227-g) packages cream cheese, softened
- ¾ cup Swerve
- 2 beaten eggs

SPECIAL EQUIPMENT:

A 12-cup muffin pan

Start by preheating the oven at 350°F (180°C) then line a muffin pan with 12 paper liners.

In a mixing bowl, mix the butter and almond meal until smooth, then spoon the mixture into the bottom of the muffin cups. Press into a flat crust.

In a mixing bowl, combine vanilla extract, cream cheese, Swerve, and eggs.

Set the electric mixer to medium, then beat the mixture until smooth.

Spoon the mixture on top of the muffin cups.

Bake in the oven until the cream cheese is nearly set in the middle, for about 17 minutes.

Remove from the oven and let the cupcakes cool.

Once cooled, refrigerate for 8 hours to overnight before serving.

STORAGE: Store in an airtight container in the fridge for up to 1 days or in the freezer for up to 1 month.

REHEAT: Microwave, covered, until the desired temperature is reached or reheat in a frying pan or air fryer / instant pot, covered, on medium.

PER SERVING

calories: 169 | fat: 16.0g | total carbs: 2.7g | fiber: 0g | protein: 3.8g

Keto Broiled Bell Pepper

Macros: Fat 66% | Proteins: 26% | Carbs 8% Prep time: 15 | Cook time: 10 minutes | Serves 4

Enjoy this tasty appetizer during any time of the day. You can add your favorite spices to taste even better.

- 2 medium bell peppers (a mix of colors)
- Kosher salt, to taste
- 1 tablespoon olive oil
- ¼ teaspoon ground cumin
- ¼ teaspoon chili powder
- 4 ounces (113 g) ground beef
- 1cup shredded Mexican blend cheese
- ¼ cup guacamole
- ¼ cup salsa
- 2 tablespoons sour cream

Cut the bell peppers through the stem into six equal parts. Remove the seeds and the stem.

Put the bell peppers in a microwave-approved dish, then add a splash of water and some salt.

Microwave while covered until the pepper pieces are pliable, for about 4 minutes.

Allow the bell peppers to cool slightly, then arrange on a baking tray lined with a foil with the cut side facing up.

In the meantime, heat the olive oil in a skillet over medium-high heat.

Add cumin and chili powder, then cook for 30 seconds while stirring.

Add ¼ teaspoon of salt, and ground beef. Sauté until the beef turns brown, for about 4 minutes.

Preheat the broiler, then spoon the beef mixture into each piece of bell pepper.

Add the cheese on top and then broil until the cheese melts, about 1 minute.

Put the guacamole and salsa on top.

Thin the sour cream out with some water and sprinkle over the peppers, then serve.

STORAGE: Store in an airtight container in the fridge for up to 3 days.

REHEAT: Microwave, covered, until the desired temperature is reached or reheat in an air fryer, covered, on medium.

PER SERVING

calories: 243 | fat: 18.1g | total carbs: 5.6g | fiber: 1.7g | protein: 15.4g

EXTRA KETO TREATS

Chocolate & Hazelnut Spread

Yields Provided: 6 Servings

Macro Counts for Each Serving:

- Fat Content: 28 g

- Total Net Carbs: 2 g

- Protein: 4 g

- Calories: 271

List of Ingredients:

- Unsalted butter (1 oz.)

- Coconut oil (.25 cup)

- Hazelnuts (5 oz.)

- Vanilla extract (1 tsp.)

- Optional: Erythritol (1 tsp.)

- Cocoa powder (2 tbsp.)

Preparation Technique:

1. Prepare the pan on the stovetop until hot. Toss in the hazelnuts and roast until golden. Let them cool slightly.
2. Arrange the nuts in a kitchen towel to rub away some of the shells.
3. Toss all of the fixings into a blender. Mix well to reach the desired consistency.

4.   Your Special Treat: Serve as a delicious and healthy dip for fresh strawberries or as a spread for rolls, waffles, or pancakes.

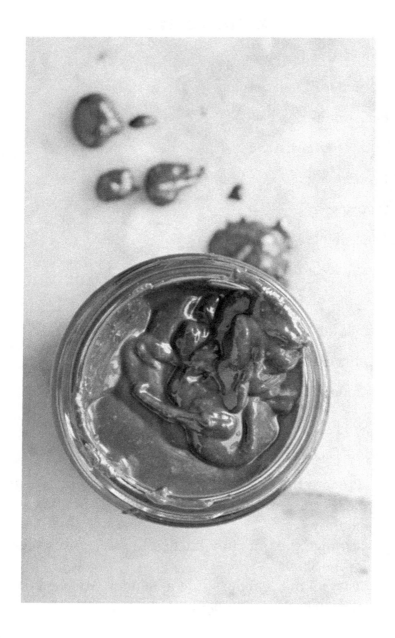

Hot Chocolate Sauce

Yields Provided: 8 Servings

Macro Counts for Each Serving:

- Total Net Carbs: 1.23 g

- Fat Content: 14.9 g

- Protein: 1.8 g

- Calories:154

List of Ingredients:

- Whipping cream (1 cup)

- Powdered Swerve Sweetener (.33 cup)

- Finely chopped unsweetened chocolate (2.5 oz.)

- Vanilla extract (.5 tsp.)

Preparation Technique:

1. Use the medium heat setting and whisk the whipping cream and sweetener until combined. Once simmering, remove from the heat.
2. Fold in the chocolate. Set aside for five minutes or until the chocolate is completely melted.
3. Whisk in the vanilla extract.
4. Drizzle over your favorite low-carb ice cream or delicious cake.

Instant Chocolate Hard Shell

Yields Provided: 32 Servings

Macro Counts for Each Serving:

- Total Net Carbs: 6.6 g

- Fat Content: 7.7 g

- Protein: 0.4 g

- Calories: 89

List of Ingredients:

- Semisweet chocolate chips (2 cups)

- Coconut oil (.66 cup)

Preparation Technique:

1. Combine the chocolate chips and coconut oil in a mixing dish.
2. Prepare using the microwave at 30-second intervals. Continue until it's creamy smooth (one to two minutes).
3. Choose a closed container and store at room temperature.

Salted Caramel Sauce

Yields Provided: 16 Servings

Macro Counts for Each Serving:

- Total Net Carbs: 0.5 g

- Fat Content: 5.5 g

- Protein: .125 g

- Calories: 52

List of Ingredients:

- Grass-fed butter - salted or unsalted (.25 cup)

- Xylitol (.25 to .5 cup)

- Heavy whipping cream (.5 cup)

- Kosher salt (.25 to .75 tsp. or to taste)

- Optional: Blackstrap molasses (1 tsp.)

Preparation Technique:

1. Add the butter to the pan using the med-low heat setting.
2. Sauté and stir about 5 minutes or until lightly browned.
3. Stir in the sweetener, heavy cream, and salt. Stir well.
4. Add in the molasses, stirring until just combined.
5. Simmer using the lowest heat setting (15 min.). Do Not Stir!
6. Taste test for sweetness. Gently add into a glass container of choice.

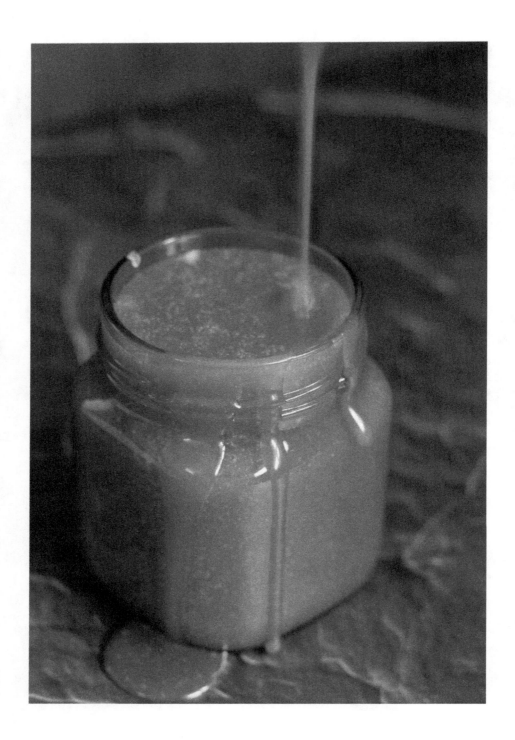

Vanilla Whipped Cream

Yields Provided: 40 Servings

Macro Counts for Each Serving:

- Total Net Carbs: 0 g
- Fat Content: 5 g
- Protein: 0 g
- Calories: 40.5

List of Ingredients:

- Heavy whipping cream (2 cups)
- Liquid stevia (2-4 tsp.) or Powder (1-2 small scoops)
- Vanilla extract (2 tsp.)

Preparation Technique:

1. Pour all of the fixings into a mixing bowl.
2. Blend until it's the consistency you like.
3. You can store this whipped cream, but it will start to liquefy.
4. Freeze it if you're not going to use it immediately.